Inspirir
and Sa
The Positive

by

Arvind Singhal
Prucia Buscell
Curt Lindberg

Bordentown, New Jersey
PlexusPress
www.plexusinstitute.org

In association with:

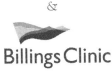

Department of Communication
The University of Texas at El Paso

&

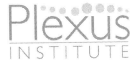

Billings, Montana

For permissions contact: info@plexusinstitute.org

PlexusPress
www.plexusinstitute.org

Design by David Hutchens www.DavidHutchens.com

ISBN: 978-0692271650

Table of Contents

This narrative is dedicated to

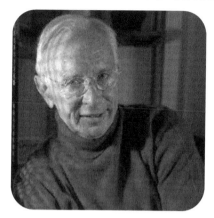

Jerry Sternin (1938-2008)
Positive Deviance Pioneer

A believer in the wisdom of all people,
he helped to unleash that wisdom to save,
and improve,
the lives of millions around the world.

Since 2005, Jerry worked with the Plexus Institute and a nationwide network of hospitals that are using the behavior change process Positive Deviance (PD) in their efforts to eliminate MRSA, a deadly pathogen that kills as many as 20,000 U.S. hospital patients each year. Three days before he passed away, Jon Lloyd, a surgeon who was Plexus Institute's Senior Clinical Advisor on MRSA prevention, visited Jerry in a Boston hospital. Jon had just returned from the recent Institute for Healthcare Improvement National Forum meeting in Nashville, where the hospitals participating in the Positive Deviance approach presented data on statistically significant reductions in MRSA rates, attributable in large measure to the PD processes that were unleashed. "Jerry was unable to speak, but almost busted my hand with a purposeful squeeze when he heard the good news," Jon reported to colleagues in the MRSA initiative. "His eyes projected great pride."

Who knows—perhaps Jerry was thinking about his fall 2006 visit to Montana, accompanied by his wife, Monique, to launch the Positive Deviance initiative at Billings Clinic.

The Sternins, along with the hundreds of frontline staff members at Billings Clinic, thus represent the real authors of the narrative that unfolds.

Preface

In one of his hundreds of guises, the mystical Sufi character Nasirudin appears on earth as a smuggler, arriving at the customs checkpoint each day leading a herd of donkeys. The customs inspector would feverishly turn the baskets hanging on the donkeys upside down to check the contents, hoping to nail Nasirudin in an act of wrongdoing. He, however, never found anything of interest, and hence had little choice but to let the smuggler go free.

Years pass, and Nasirudin's legend as a smuggler grew while the inspector grew ever more frustrated. One day, after Nasirudin and the inspector had retired from their respective occupations, their paths crossed. The former inspector pleaded, "Tell me, Nasirudin. What were you smuggling?"

"Donkeys," Nasirudin said.

Nasirudin's donkey story holds important lessons for social, organizational and behavioral change practitioners. Often the solutions to highly intractable problems, whether in communities or organizations, stare us in the face, but remain unseen. To discover these invisible, in-house, innovative practices, we need to engage the Positive Deviance (PD) approach to social, organizational, and individual change.

The PD approach is based on the premise that every community has individuals or groups whose uncommon behaviors and strategies enable them to find better solutions to problems than their peers although everyone has the same challenges and access to the same resources (Pascale, Sternin, & Sternin, 2010; Singhal & Dura, 2009). Consider a physician who makes rounds on patients in a way that he visits the ones with MRSA infections last. Consider a nursing assistant who has developed the ability to confront surgeons about to enter isolation rooms without taking the required precautions and convince them to wash their hands and put on gowns and gloves. In both cases, these small, non-normative behaviors reduce the risk of spreading deadly infections, saving patients' lives. However, such behaviors are ordinarily invisible to others, and especially to expert change agents. The physician and the nursing assistant in these cases represent "deviants" because their uncommon behaviors are not the norm; they are "positive" deviants because they have found ways to effectively address the problem, while most others have not (Singhal, 2013; Singhal, Buscell, & Lindberg, 2010). The PD approach relies on unearthing the wisdom that lies hidden with "unusual suspects," and amplifying it in a process that leads to sustainable organizational and community transformation.

This work analyzes a remarkable case of the application of PD to dramatically improve the quality of patient care and reduce hospital-acquired infections in Billings Clinic, Billings, Montana. While the present authors have in part documented the Billings Clinic case (see our previous volume Singhal, Buscell, & Lindberg, 2010), the nuances and subtleties of this still-unfolding story at Billings Clinic inspire us to share it more fully in this monograph. We believe that you will find this updated story of PD at Billings Clinic intriguing and interesting.

In his Foreword to our 2010 book, *Inviting Everyone: Healing Healthcare through Positive Deviance*, Peter Block, the noted organizational change author and practitioner, observed (quoted in Singhal, Buscell, & Lindberg, 2010, p. vii):

"Positive Deviance is much more radical than even its practitioners imagine. Radical in the best sense, it is joining a new field of inquiry, which might be called communal transformation."

We organize the story of this communal transformation at Billings Clinic in three sections:

- **Section 1:** *Making the Invisible Visible: Learning to See and Stop MRSA at Billings Clinic*
  This section documents the early years (2005 to 2009) of the Billings experience with the Positive Deviance approach, focusing on the cultural transformation of frontline staff in reducing hospital-acquired infections (notably MRSA) and in improving patient safety and quality.

- **Section 2:** *The Postscript: A Quality Cascade*
  This section documents the unfolding, cascading, and constant improvements in patient safety (from 2009 to 2014) at Billings Clinic, building on the cultural shifts engendered by Positive Deviance. It also documents the expansion of PD to address other intractable and complex clinical issues such as expanding use of palliative care and management of hypertension, diabetes and pain.

- **Section 3:** *Resources on Positive Deviance*
  This section is directed to readers who wish to engage more deeply with the scholarly literature on the Positive Deviance approach. It is comprised of over 100 peer-reviewed publications that address a wide variety of complex social problems, including improving patient safety in healthcare settings, and a variety of other public health issues, such as decreasing malnutrition, enhancing reproductive health, and protecting children from exploitation.

We invite you to engage with this remarkable story of organizational and communal change at Billings Clinic, where an actionable approach called Positive Deviance is saving patients' lives.

Arvind Singhal
Prucia Buscell
Curt Lindberg

Section I

Making the Invisible Visible
Learning to See and Stop MRSA
at Billings Clinic

This section documents the early years (2005 to 2009) of the Billings Clinic experience with the Positive Deviance approach, focusing on the cultural transformation of frontline staff in reducing hospital-acquired infections (notably MRSA) and in improving patient safety and quality.

Making the Invisible Visible

"It's as if we are in a canoe paddling across an ocean toward No-MRSA land. We have a general sense of direction. We have gained some oars. But we need more rowers. While not everyone is in the boat yet, enough are to make a difference."

–Carlos Arce, director,
organizational and leadership development

Microbes and memes—the ideas and activities that are the intellectual equivalent of genes— share common traits. They are self-replicating entities that multiply and spread, impacting human communities with unpredictable waves of change for good and ill. They are also invisible to the naked eye.

With perseverance and sharpened perception, however, the invisible can be illuminated. Just as the ripples in the wake of the canoe make forward progress discernable, other evidence of things unseen guides and colors the vision of the travelers to No MRSA Land.

Billings Clinic
Infection Control Surveillance Report
MRSA Healthcare-associated Infections Incidence rates

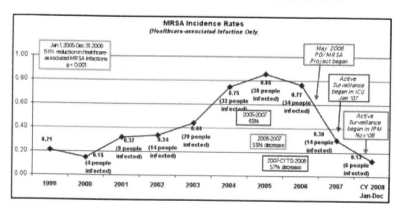

Infection rates for the deadly pathogen Methicillin resistant *Staphylococcus aureus*, also known as MRSA, have been rising in most U.S. hospitals. But the sharp decline in infection rates at Billings Clinic, documented by carefully gathered data, gives evidence that an innovative prevention effort has been abundantly productive.

Billings Clinic, a not for profit, multi-specialty group practice and 272-bed hospital in Billings, Montana, reduced housewide health-care-associated MRSA infections by 84% in the past two and a half years, a spectacular achievement especially as infection rates had increased relentlessly in previous years.

CDC analysts determined that Billings Clinic has achieved a highly statistically significant decline—meaning it is highly likely that the drop is associated with the MRSA-fighting initiative, and did not happen by chance. An analysis of the data, by John Jernigan, MD, MS, the CDC's MRSA expert, and colleagues at the CDC and Billings, was presented at the March 2009 meeting of the Society for Healthcare Epidemiology of America. Interestingly, as MRSA rates dropped at Billings and two other hospitals, the hospitals also saw a decline in the percentage of *Staph aureus* infections caused by the Methicillin resistant variety, signifying that hospitals can make headway in the fight against drug-resistant superbugs.

"This hospital has apparently dramatically reduced the risk of acquiring MRSA for its patients, and that's a goal we hope every hospital would try for," Dr. Jernigan said of Billings Clinic. Referring to the recent analysis, he said, "These extremely encouraging findings add to a growing body of evidence that hospitals can make a difference in their endemic MRSA rates, and further might be able to improve the chances that patients have the best possible treatment options available. It shows that hospitals can make an important difference in antimicrobial resistance even at a time when the availability of new antibiotics has stagnated."

Healthcare-Acquired Infection's Daily Toll

"We are wading upstream in an ever widening and deepening MRSA river."

—Jon Lloyd, MD, senior clinical advisor, Plexus Institute

Hospital acquired infections (HAIs) kill some 100,000 Americans each year[i] – more than AIDS, breast cancer, and auto accidents combined. Methicillin resistant *Staphylococcus aureus* (MRSA) is associated with the deaths of 20,000 hospital patients a year and the illness and suffering of thousands more.

Among hospital-acquired infections, MRSA infections increased 32-fold between 1976 and 2004, and the U.S., shamefully, is second only to Japan in national MRSA prevalence.[ii] Some 100 million Americans (one in three) carry the bacterium *Staph aureus*[iii] and nearly three million carry the drug-resistant strain that cannot be treated by Methicillin and other commonly used antibiotics. Most U.S. hospitals (up to 95 percent) do not know which patients, at the time of admission, are MRSA carriers.[iv] Knowing their status is vital because some 30 percent of all MRSA carriers will develop a serious MRSA infection.

MRSA is a preventable infection. Adherence to hand hygiene, gloving, and gowning protocols can drastically reduce the incidence of MRSA transmission. However, hand hygiene studies in U.S. hospitals, conducted between 1994 and 2000, showed pitiful adherence rates: from 29 percent to 48 percent. In other words,

Jennifer Mellgren-Blackford, MT (ASCP), CIC, quality specialist in infection control, recalled that she and colleagues had been shocked when they first saw the declining rates. Dr. David Graham, one of two infectious disease physicians, agrees. "I don't know how you could not be surprised by these results," he said. "We were all looking for ways they could be wrong. How did we get here?" Nancy Iversen, director of patient safety and infection control, sums up the impact: "The declining graph is more than mere lines etched on paper. It tells the story of lives saved, pain avoided, and suffering reduced."

most encounters between healthcare providers and patients in U.S. carry a high risk of MRSA transmission. Hygeia, the Greek goddess of being well and preventing sickness would be seething with anger.

People expect hospitals to be safe environments, not transmission vectors of deadly pathogens. They expect doctors and nurses and therapists to cure and heal, not harm. What does it mean for unsuspecting patients (and their families) when these healers do not wash their hands, or are too busy to properly gown and glove?

Despite policy mandates, educational campaigns, health quality improvement projects, system redesigns, and adherence report cards, MRSA infection rates in U.S. healthcare facilities continue to sky-

rocket. The focus of MRSA prevention initiatives, to date, has been top-down, expert-driven, technological fixes. However, non-adherence to hygiene procedures is a behavioral problem, governed by social and cultural norms. Surprisingly, highly-educated care-givers, especially those cloaked in scientific armor, allow MRSA pathogens to slip by.

For unsuspecting citizens, such lapses are inexcusable.

The Billings Clinic MRSA reduction has profound public health implications. MRSA has become a national story, and an October 2007 story in the *Journal of the American Medical Association* reported that 85 percent of all MRSA cases originate in healthcare settings. Evidence now shows rising hospital-acquired infections (HAIs), considered for years as an intractable problem, can be overcome. And not by technical directives, punitive action, or pharmaceutical intervention, but by tapping the inherent wisdom of the organization's frontline staff.

> ## *"We exist temporarily through what we take, but we live forever through what we give."*

Billings Clinic's vision of sharing and caring.

For too long, the U.S. healthcare industry has been too focused on fixing errors and preoccupied with correcting what is wrong. The Clinic's approach to MRSA prevention focuses on what works, believing that among its vast pool of employees—doctors, nursing staff, housekeepers, therapists, patient transporters, technicians, pastors, social workers, and support staff—there are individuals who practice certain simple yet uncommon behaviors that prevent MRSA transmission. For instance, in doing his hospital rounds, a Billings Clinic physician purposely sees his MRSA patients last—a simple practice that greatly reduces the risk of transmitting MRSA. An ICU nurse disinfects the patient's side rails several times throughout her shift to keep MRSA from being picked up and spread to other patients.

In the new lexicon of the Clinic, these individuals are "positive deviants." They are "deviants" because their behaviors are not the norm and "positive" as they model the desirable MRSA-prevention behaviors.

So, the Billings' MRSA-reduction story is about an organization tapping its readily-available resource to unleash innovative ways of preventing transmissions.

Join us on a visit to Billings Clinic.

Billings Clinic:
A Bastion of Healing

L ocated in the beautiful Yellowstone River Valley, Billings Clinic sits in the city of Billings,[v] a couple of miles from the "Rimrocks" (or Rims)—the sandstone cliffs enclosing the city. Several million years ago, the Rims were a plain sandy beach before the Yellowstone River began to carve the topography into valleys and gorges. The Battle of the Little Bighorn, in which the combined forces of Lakota and Northern Cheyenne Indians defeated the Seventh Cavalry of the U.S. Army, happened here in 1876. A few years later the valley was being settled as a railroad town, and acquired the name Billings, after Fredrick H. Billings,[vi] the President of the Northern Pacific Railroad. Two main commercial streets were built in the mid-1880s along the railroad tracks and named Montana and Minnesota Avenues. The main Billings Clinic complex sits a few blocks north of Montana Avenue.

Billings Clinic, the largest employer in Billings, with 3,500 employees, is a multi-specialty group practice of more than 250 physicians and 65 non-physician providers. Patterned after the famous Mayo Clinic in Rochester, MN, Billings Clinic is a not-for-profit organization, governed by the community, with physicians in leadership positions. In 2007, the Clinic's revenues were $475 million, and while its operating margins amounted to three percent, the institution had funneled some 11 percent of its revenues—about $48 million—back into the community, including contributions to charity care, subsidized health services, and community health initiatives.

A boldly painted wall on the main floor captures the Billings Clinic's explicit vision of "Sharing and Caring." It reads: "We exist temporarily through what we take, but we live forever through what we give."

Walking the corridors of Billings Clinic, the institution's vision of caring plays out in multiple fractal patterns, each reinforcing the other. On a bulletin board in a staff restroom, hung a two-sided, hand-written patient letter. It said:

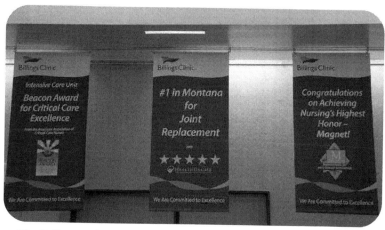

"I wanted to take this opportunity to let you know how much I appreciate the kind; compassionate; and efficient care I have received here. The worst encounter I have had here with any of the staff has been at worst; delightful. I wish I could go around and thank everyone for making a stressful and traumatic event in my life, the pleasant experience it has been......"

There is a simple but deep explanation for why a discharged patient might be motivated to write this letter. Billings Clinic has personal service expectations for every interaction that its staff has with a patient, guest, superior, or colleague. We observed and experienced the "Ten Foot Circle" service expectation, that is, mindfully acknowl-

The Billings Clinic vision is to be number one in quality, patient safety, and service

edging those who come into one's physical proximity. Staff members initiated polite conversation when riding elevators, and habitually held the door open for others. A phone is answered in four rings or less, and permission is sought before putting "Mr. Jones" on hold. Patients are referred to by name, not as "the diabetic in Room 223."

Billings Clinic's vision is not small: By 2010, it aims "to be recognized as the healthcare organization providing the best clinical quality, patient safety and service experience in the nation." The many kudos flags hanging in the main conference room, and the glass obelisk in the cafeteria recognizing Billings' Magnet designation for nursing excellence, suggest that Billings Clinic is not all talk. This healthcare organization relentlessly walks the talk.

Change from Within:
Harnessing Positive Deviance[vi]

Billings Clinic's MRSA-prevention mantra is anchored on the Positive Deviance (PD) approach, a social and organizational change strategy that enables communities to discover the wisdom they already have, and then to act on it.[vii]

PD gained recognition in the work of Tufts nutrition professor Marian Zeitlin when she began focusing on why some children in poor communities were better nourished than others.[viii] Zeitlin argued that change agents should identify what's going right in a community in order to amplify that, as opposed to looking for what's going wrong in a community and fixing it.[ix]

The late Jerry Sternin,[x] who directed the Positive Deviance Ini-

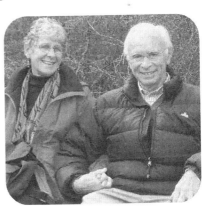

Monique and Jerry Sternin

Healing a Person, Not a Body

"What can I do for you?" asked a Billings nurse of a terminally-ill patient.

"Would you wheel me to the fish pond?" he whispered.

Gazing at the trout for what seemed like an hour, he murmured: "Now I can die in peace."

After a pause, he smiled at the nurse and said: "Fishing was my first love!"

During our three-day visit to Billings Clinic, we heard the above story twice, narrated by two different people, each rendering a slightly different treatment. However, on both occasions it evoked the same reflection – a line from the movie, Patch Adams:

"You treat a disease you win, you lose. You treat a person, you win no matter what the outcome."

Billings Clinic's Healing Environment Program combines the science and technology of medicine with the aesthetics of the arts. Outside the main building, sprawls a healing garden with various plants, rocks, a flowing water stream, and an exhibit about the Deaconess Billings Clinic (the Clinic's former name). One slate discusses the Deaconess philosophy of nursing—treat the whole person—and shows a figure of the Lady with the Lamp, Florence Nightingale. We learn that Nurse Nightingale, who many believe was the second most famous Victorian in England after Queen Victoria herself, was trained in the Deaconess system of training.

Billings' focus on healing the person now makes even more sense.

We sit in the cafeteria, sipping Java coffee. The soothing sound of a baby grand piano comes on. Adjacent to the cafeteria is the pharmacy. The counter is adorned by dozens of flower bouquets and plants.

"Ah, being healed as one waits on one's prescription," we muse.

Walking the corridors of the Clinic, we notice the original and collected works of art. Nancy Iversen, our escort, points to a subtle, exquisite, monochromatic landscape titled "Winter Dusk and Big Sky"—a rendering of the Big Sky Montana country. The painting is an original Russell Chatham, a world-renowned Montana lithographer whose patrons include Hollywood legends Peter Fonda and Jack Nicholson. Another painting is by Ben Steele, a former Billings Clinic patient and a famed Montana artist, who survived the Bataan Death March in 1942 off the Bataan Peninsula, Philippines. His sketches of the 60-mile long Bataan Death March and Japanese army atrocities, drawn from memory after surviving the ordeal, are well-known internationally.

In the inpatient surgical unit sits a traffic light type contraption: A noise meter that turns red when the decibels go up. Most of the hospital is designated as a noise-free zone. In a "healing" room, right next to patients undergoing chemotherapy, we notice a stack of fragrant candles, incense sticks, and an inviting massage chair. An RCA boom box sits on a table, playing a Tranquility Collection of forest rain and wood-wind melodies.

Heal a person, no matter what the outcome, you win. Billings Clinic = Healing.

tiative at Tufts University with his wife and collaborator, Monique, built on Zeitlin's ideas to organize various PD-centered social change interventions around the world. The Sternins used PD to address such diverse and intractable problems as reintegrating returned abductees and child mothers in conflict-ridden Northern Uganda, eliminating female genital cutting in Egypt, curbing trafficking of young girls in Indonesia, increasing school retention rates in Argentina, and higher levels of condom use among commercial sex workers in Vietnam and Myanmar.

In 1991, as Director of Save the Children in Vietnam, Mr. Sternin was asked by government officials to create an effective, large-scale program to combat child malnutrition, and to demonstrate results within six months. More than 65 percent of all children living in the

Vietnamese villages were malnourished at the time. The task seemed impossible.

Building on Zeitlin's ideas, the Sternins sought poor families who had managed to avoid malnutrition without access to any special resources. They were the positive deviants (PDs). They helped the communities to discover that mothers in these families collected tiny shrimps and crabs from paddy fields, and added those with sweet potato greens to their children's meals.[xi] Also, these PD mothers were feeding their children three to four times a day, rather than the customary twice a day. PD mothers were also more likely to actively feed their children by hand, in contrast to most mothers who just placed the rice bowl in front of their children.

"We dance around in a ring and suppose, while the secret sits in the middle and knows."

–Robert Frost

The Sternins helped the community to design a program whereby community members could emulate the positive deviants. Mothers whose children were malnourished were asked to forage for shrimps, crabs, and sweet potato greens, and in the company of other mothers, learned to cook new recipes that their children ate right there. Within weeks, mothers could see their children becoming healthier.

After the pilot study, which lasted two years, malnutrition had decreased by an amazing 85 percent in the communities where PD was implemented. Over the next several years, the PD intervention became a nationwide program in Vietnam. The meme replicated through families and villages, helping over 2.2 million people, including over 500,000 children, improve their nutritional status.[xii]

The PD approach emphasizes hands-on learning and focuses on actionable behaviors.[xiii] It subscribes to the philosophy: "It is easier to act your way into a new way of thinking than to think your way into a new way of acting."[xiv] In healthcare contexts, PD bridges the gap between what healthcare workers know and what they do. They know infection control protocols, but they don't follow them consistently. PD processes enable front line staff to identify practices that already work, and to discover for themselves the best ways to implement them.

PD Comes to Billings

In the summer of 2004, Billings CEO Nick Wolter, MD attended a workshop in Durham, NH, sponsored by Plexus Institute[xv] and the Harvard Interfaculty Program for Health Systems Improvement in Cambridge, MA. In this workshop, Jerry Sternin made an impromptu 15-minute presentation on Positive Deviance, narrating the Vietnam story. In a follow-up conversation with Dr. Wolter, Mr. Sternin emphasized that PD was especially suited to address intractable problems. The next day, Mr.

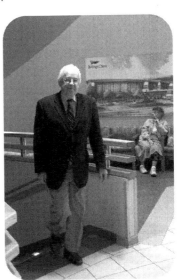

Sternin was invited to lead a discussion on how PD could be applied to one of the most intractable problems in U.S. hospitals: adherence to hand hygiene. Several hospital CEOs, including Billings Clinic's Nick Wolter[xvi] participated.

When Dr. Wolter returned to Billings, he told a senior staff meeting: "This [PD] might be a 'good' idea."

Jon Ness, Chief Operating Office of Billings, says: "When Nick says it is a 'good' idea, it is a code word for 'let's try it'."

Mr. Ness recalls: "Nick knew that when it came to hand hygiene adher-

Nick Wolter, MD, Billings Clinic CEO. His windowless office is in the basement. "The mission of administration is to serve," he noted.

23

ence and other patient safety issues, we had plateaued with technical solutions and fixes. The fabric of leadership here is high achievement....Nick breathes quality and safety....so it was our obligation to support innovative approaches."[xvii]

The principles of infection control have been known for ages. Hand hygiene and contact isolation precautions were established in the mid-nineteenth century by Ignaz Semmelweis, a Hungarian doctor who while working as an obstetrician in Vienna's General Hospital, became intrigued by a puzzling statistic: the hospital ward in which obstetricians delivered babies had three times the maternal mortality rate compared to the ward where the midwives were in charge. Semmelweis noticed that the obstetricians dissected cadavers in the morning and then, in the afternoon, examined their patients with bare unwashed hands. Hypothesizing that infectious agents were spread to women patients by the physicians, Semmelweis[xviii] implemented more rigorous hand-washing and scrubbing procedure in the doctors' ward, most notably with chloride-of-lime solutions, a powerful antiseptic. Infections dropped precipitously—from 17 percent of all patients to one percent.

Despite this scientific knowledge, compliance with hand hygiene protocols among most healthcare workers remains less than 50 percent. Gowns, gloves, and consistent hand hygiene are often viewed as a time consuming nuisance. The insight that knowledge does not change behavior was the reason why Billings Clinic was paying more and more attention to addressing the "how" of behavior change. The "how" was Positive Deviance.

Nick Wolter sent Nancy Iversen, the director of patient safety, to a workshop on Positive Deviance, conducted by Jerry and Monique Sternin, in Boston in July 2005. Ms. Iversen, inspired by how people at Waterbury Hospital in Connecticut had achieved early success with using PD for medication reconciliation, was eager to start PD at Billings Clinic.

The next year, Billings Clinic became one of the six beta site health-care systems that took part in a Plexus Institute-led MRSA Prevention Partnership.[xix] These beta sites agreed to tackle MRSA as a behavioral and social problem using Positive Deviance as the driving approach. In late summer 2006, a Billings Clinic team led by Ms. Iversen, visited the Veterans Health Administration Pittsburgh Healthcare System (VAPHS), a sister beta site that had implemented PD some months previously, and had some lessons to share.[xx]

In spring 2006, the Plexus team that included Jerry and Monique Sternin and Keith McCandless had come to Billings Clinic for the PD MRSA kick-off event. The Sternins' visit generated both enthusiasm and skepticism. However, with CEO Nick Wolter's backing, and Billings Clinic's commitment to be a beta site partner on the Plexus Institute-led MRSA Prevention Partnership, the PD process began to roll.

Keith McCandless and Joelle Everett, two highly accomplished organizational change consultants, and Monique Sternin, were coaches for the Billings PD MRSA initiative. Just after the kickoff event staff who were interested in working on stopping MRSA infections met to begin.

As 2006 was coming to a close, Billings Clinic had initiated a concerted MRSA prevention program consisting of active surveillance, culturing of patients admitted to the Intensive

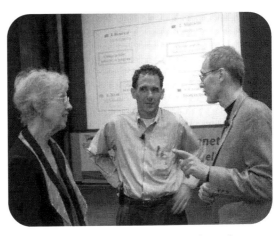

Coaches Joelle Everett (left) and Keith Mc-Candless (right) with Carlos Arce, director, organizational and leadership development at Billings Clinic

Care Unit (ICU), contact precautions for any patient in the hospital known to be colonized or infected with MRSA, hand hygiene, and hospital-wide implementation of the Positive Deviance approach to improve adherence to infection control practices.

The first step at Billings Clinic was a rigorous effort to get a baseline on MRSA prevalence. A prevalence study on all hospital patients and 300 volunteer healthcare workers was conducted in the fall of 2006. The MRSA prevalence rates for patients at Billings Clinic were in line with national averages: just under eight percent for patients using traditional culturing techniques, and 12 percent using rapid testing methods. For the employee study, they found some seven percent overall prevalence, eight percent among the nursing staff, and 17 percent among physicians, nurse practitioners, and physician assistants. The licensed providers, especially male physicians, had the highest MRSA colonization rates.

It was an important step. "When we first started, there was a misconception that everyone has MRSA, I have it, others have it, so what's the point of this and why have isolation?" recalled Dania Block, RN, clinical coordinator of the ICU "The prevalence study showed not everyone does have it."

Jerry Sternin used to explain that PD is "bathed in data." In time, the staff at Billings Clinic would become ardent measurers, and proficient interpreters of new data. But scientific and quantitative data can flow in unexpected ways, leave shadows, create tributaries and carry psychic impact. The commitment to active surveillance in pilot units meant screening every patient with a nasal swab on admission, transfer and discharge. That meant vastly more work for nursing staff and laboratory, and burgeoning record keeping. Hand hygiene and adherence to other infection control protocols would be tracked and recorded, and supplies, purchases and usage documented. Routines would change, rhythms of the workplace would be altered, and some habits would have to be unlearned. Would it be worth it? Ms. Iversen

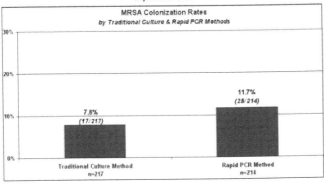

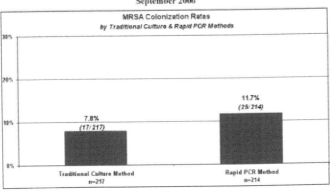

Study showing licensed providers
with highest MRSA colonization rates

recalls Dr. Wolter had said, "Go ahead and stir things up. We're behind you."

It was a turbulent beginning. ICU Manager Michaela Harakal had been very enthusiastic. "We just jumped in with both feet and no life jacket, and it was my fault," she said in retrospect. "I said we have to do this in ICU. I had not thought about the impact on staff and our work processes.

"Everyone had been through staff orientation about what PD was, what MRSA was, and how we could impact it, and everyone was on board" she continued. "When the work started, and we started isolating infected patients and carriers, it threw the nurses for a loop… It was just so hard. We couldn't get all the processes down, and we couldn't get certain staff to buy into the processes of gowning and gloving."

"Don't be buffaloed by experts and elites. Experts often possess more data than judgment. Elites can become so inbred that they produce hemophiliacs who bleed to death as soon as they are nicked by the real world."

–Colin Powell, former Secretary of State, retired Army general

Was it necessary to put on gowns and gloves every time a person entered an isolation room to answer a call light, or check a pump? What if you didn't plan to touch the patient? Some staff members wanted to find ways to avoid the gear, such as requiring it only if one crossed a line taped on the floor. "Then we had another presentation from the Infection Control department, showing how long bacteria can live on surfaces, how it gets all over the room, and how even if you don't touch the patient, you will touch something," Ms. Block said. "That was a turning point for us. "

Nurses got past that hurdle, and Ms. Harakal and Ms. Block remember working to help physicians get past the same hurdle. "When physicians went into an isolation room without gown and gloves, the nurses wouldn't let them out until they had at least washed their hands," Ms. Harakal said. "One of our directors went into a room with gown and gloves, but didn't wash his hands on the way out. Dania is tall— 6' 1" and she just stood in the doorway with a bottle of GelSan. He looked up at her…then cleaned his hands. It was pretty funny."

Some resistance was more strident. Ms. Harakal recalls that when a nurse handed one surgeon a gown, he balled it up and threw it at her. "He was a friend of one our intensivists," she said. "I asked him to please talk to his friend and tell him that isn't something we do here."

Ms. Block and Ms. Harakal say doctors, including a disbelieving surgeon, are consistently using proper isolation gear now. "A year ago, I'd say it was only fifty-fifty," Ms. Block said.

Dr. David Graham and fellow Infectious Disease Physician Dr. Camilla Saberhagen say physicians now view gowns, gloves and isolation differently, as things that simply have to be done rather than matters of choice. But they agree physician behavior is hard to change, and that Positive Deviance was initially viewed with suspicion. Physician education fosters autonomy and independent judgment, both said. As Dr. Graham puts it, "You're put through a wringer to decide things for yourself, and if you start doubting your decisions you often become ineffective at what you're supposed to be doing."

"When you're trained in a solitary role as the ultimate decision maker, many find it harder to embrace team concepts," said Dr. Saberhagen. "When you start talking about PD, for many, that challenges the foundations of what they think of as problem solving. It's a different paradigm.

"I know some of the physicians who responded negatively when a nurse would hand them a gown and gloves," she continues, "and they are really very nice people." She adds that the PD process includes meetings, which doctors try to avoid. She and Dr. Graham hopes more physicians will "come on board."

Dr. Saberhagen says her own doubts began to melt when she heard discussions among staff members who had been involved with PD. She was struck by how intense they were about helping with patient care, safety and quality. She had worked at Billings from 1999 to

2004, left, and then returned in April 2008 when the PD process was underway. "When I was here the first time, we were struggling with hand hygiene and isolation, and how to get it all to work," she said. "When I came back, there was a very different tone. The staff felt empowered to effect change. They were willing to speak up about what they felt was right. Many already knew what they were supposed to do. But it seemed they now really took ownership, they weren't just following rules and policies. And I think PD is the first thing I've seen that can bring about change in multiple areas by getting the right players involved."

Much has been written about how to effect change in various industries, Dr. Saberhagen reflects, and managers can supply numbers and quality indicators. "But if you want to know what works, you have to ask the frontline people," she said. "That's where the rubber meets the road. Getting things to happen on the front lines is a huge problem in healthcare."

A recent success has been data showing a 14 week period with no MRSA transmissions in the ICU, and the admission and discharge swabbing rates have been better than 90 percent for months. "That gives everyone the drive to go ahead," Ms. Harakal said. "Our next step is to eradicate MRSA. We want to get to zero."

The data that is so helpful now didn't come easily. For one thing, it takes time to gather information that proves whether something is working, and as Dr. Saberhagen notes, physicians are attuned to immediate results. In addition, nurses and physicians questioned the validity of the MRSA test results. Bob Merchant, MD, a pulmonary and intensive care physician, found that in the 22 bed ICU, traditional lab tests identified only eight patients with MRSA while a more expensive test identified 12. "What good are the tests, if they don't identify all cases?" he asked. The lab staff thought current tests were accurate, and demanded proof to show otherwise. "Never say 'prove it' to an ICU nurse," Ms. Harakal declared. "We did a two week study, and Dania saw that samples were being retrieved and sent to the lab properly, and we found that by changing culture mediums, we got more accurate results." Paula Jackson, MT (ASCP), lead microbiologist, and her team confirmed that different tests produced varying results. After conversations with other beta sites and learning they were using specialized agar, she agreed to adopt this inexpensive and more specific test. But it took nearly a year to reach consensus on testing, and that was not the only issue that took time.

Many physicians remained dubious. Disagreements about the early PD effort were not uncommon. Ms. Harakal notes that PD is initially hard for people accustomed to scientific, evidence-based ways of thinking. Ms. Block, who describes herself as a "true believer" now, commented, "In the beginning I thought the PD approach was too touchy-feely." Lu Byrd, chief nursing officer, recalls that conducting active MRSA surveillance was a challenge that caused tensions. Swabbing all patients on admission and discharge seemed to be an elusive goal, and at one point the discharge swabbing rate dropped. "The problem was we were relying on computers to give the task to nurses," she recalls, and they weren't getting the message. Dr. Merchant had responded that technology alone doesn't solve all human problems, adding, "I have never seen 100 percent hand hygiene. ...and there was low communication between administration and staff in the beginning. But that has improved."

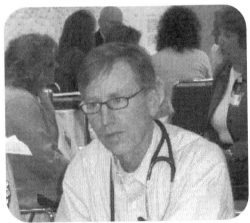

The ICU twice rebelled over data, and wanted out of the program. "We had a nice program on

Robert Merchant, MD, wanted more sensitive data.

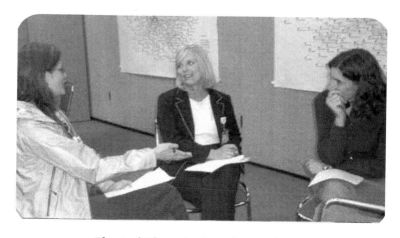

Physical Therapist Jennifer Leachman,
Jennifer Mellgren-Blackford, quality specialist in infection control,
and Camilla Saberhagen, MD

paper, but we weren't connecting with people the right way," Ms. Iversen said in retrospect. Weekly reports were being sent to leadership, and at one point, some transmissions had occurred, and compliance on hand hygiene and isolation precautions seemed to be down. ICU staff members took exception to the data and its interpretation. Dr. Merchant, sensing their frustration, convened a gathering to discuss whether to continue the program in ICU, and if so, how to seek commitment by all. This was at a time that many staff members still questioned whether the extra work was justified. "I was one of the people standing in front of a group saying we didn't want to do this any more," Ms. Harakal said.

Then a door cracked open. Ms. Byrd recalls a meeting with ICU staff and leadership where she and Ms. Iversen displayed charts showing a dramatic drop in MRSA infections. Both knew the power of information made visible. A staff nurse asked when they could quit this unwieldy project. Upon seeing the charts, the ICU staff answered their own question: "Never."

That was in October, 2007, when the ICU leadership, Ms. Iversen and Ms. Byrd met to continue the PD MRSA discussions and try to soothe tensions. "The medical staff in that unit didn't call themselves champions—they rejected that term as a buzz word," Ms. Byrd recalled. "Pulmonary did co-develop a program with ICU. It just wasn't painless or easy."

Carlos Arce, director of organizational development, was part of the PD MRSA Partnership, and was drawn to the project because of its novelty and the opportunity to contribute directly to patient care. He admits he wearied of the data disputes and math wars. "Data can be used in distracting ways," he observed. "It's as though the germs have figured out that humans are inclined to argue over these figures. The departments that had the most heated arguments seemed to demonstrate the least progress. But we had to continue our work."

"People look to Dr. Merchant as a leader," continued Mr. Arce. "He is an example of someone who is trusted in the organization because of how he interacts with people....We had to make sure we had healthy relationships so that we could address difficult topics and not have a defensive response. It's part of our journey around service."

Peggy Wharton, RN, MS, vice president of clinic operations, reflects on another data issue—the elusive quest for unequivocal accuracy. "Physicians will make changes if they are presented with applicable data that demonstrates the need for change. Physicians want perfection, have high standards and expect everyone to function at a high level. Data helps drive their decisions."

Keith McCandless, a consultant who helped Billings persevere with the PD MRSA initiative, posed a "wicked question"—the kind of question that dislodges self-fulfilling prophesies: *How is it that without complete data or evidence, we are getting great results from our prevention efforts?*

Mr. Arce suggests some answers. One involves a Billings culture that demonstrates adaptability. Perhaps, he suggests, it has to do with

Making History

Shelley Fritel, Data Analyst, Quality Resources, has a felicitous memory of one of those rare, flashing "Eureka" moments. It suddenly struck her that something very new and different was happening, and that Billings Clinic was poised to make history.

Ms. Fritel had accompanied Billings Clinic director of patient safety and infection control, Nancy Iversen, and Jennifer Mellgren-Blackwell, quality specialist in infection control, to a training session conducted by the CDC in Atlanta. Participants were learning to use a new MRSA surveillance system. It is the first of its kind in the country, and it came about through an unusual collaboration. Trish Perl, MD, professor of medicine, pathology and epidemiology at Johns Hopkins Hospital, worked with infection control professionals at the Plexus PD MRSA beta site hospitals in collaboration with John Jernigan, MD, the CDC's acting deputy chief of prevention and response, and his CDC colleagues. The new surveillance system lets beta site hospitals collect and submit uniform data on MRSA infections. It is now part of the CDC's National Healthcare Safety Network (NHSN) and available to any hospital in the U.S. that wants to use it. Addressing the group, Dr. Jernigan described the ravages of MRSA in U.S. healthcare, and explained the value to hospitals providing the data: they can evaluate their own progress in infection fighting over time and learn how their efforts compare with similar healthcare organizations.

"I still get goose bumps when I think about it," Ms. Fritel said recently. "What has really stayed with me is that we are making history. MRSA is on the rise, and if we can reverse that, we really are making a contribution."

Ms. Fritel is in charge of the data base where the Billings Clinic information on MRSA data is maintained. She takes enormous pride in the numbers that show an 84 percent drop in MRSA infections. Her department collects data on active MRSA surveillance, infections, transmissions, contact precaution and hand hygiene compliance. She prepares graphs so that data is transformed into information the staff can use to act on the results.

For Ms. Fritel, the fight against MRSA is passionate and personal. Her son, Garth, now a pharmacist in Spokane, Washington, had back surgery at Billings Clinic in July, 2002. He got a MRSA infection, needed a second surgery, and endured a slow and agonizing recovery. He struggled through his first semester in Pharmacy school in a fog of pain and medication.

During Garth's MRSA ordeal, Ms. Fritel was a supervisor in patient accounts. She had trained as a nurse, studied psychology, and served as a tech staffer in a state program to help emergency patients arrange regular care. She didn't know Nancy Iversen then, but when she heard about the data analyst job in 2002 she jumped at the chance.

She was gratified to discover she would help with data vital in fighting the infection that had afflicted her son. She is enthusiastic about the potential for new developments in data collection and use. One innovation developed by the CDC for this initiative, for example, is a surrogate measure that enables hospitals to quickly evaluate the impact of PD or other change efforts on their MRSA rate. Because the new measure is based on the results of positive clinical cultures that are already stored in the existing laboratory data bases, CDC analysts are now able to electronically extract data that show long term trends so that changes before and after an intervention can be identified.

"I am proud of our system, and working in this department, and being a part of this project, that is dear to my heart," Ms. Fritel said. "It hasn't been easy. A lot of people didn't buy into this right away. But Nancy just kept on pushing. People here are the best. I feel so lucky to come to work every day and love what I do, and my son is thrilled that we are taking on MRSA and reducing it." Years later sitting in a Discovery and Action dialogue, when the ICU asked if they could pull out of the project, she was able to speak up on behalf of patients and their families. She remembers asking "have any ICU staff experienced MRSA? If so, you wouldn't want to stop".

Montana's Western traditions of openness, pioneering and a willingness to depart from convention. "There is a catch 22 in the data debate," he mused.

Take active surveillance: do the results justify the time and effort of MRSA testing with a nasal swab for every patient upon admission, transfer and discharge? "If you wait until the data is in, you do nothing, and generate no new data. Another possibility is to try everything, and see what happens to the data. I think what made us able to do that is a spirit of innovation, risk taking, or lack of hierarchy, and ultimately our willingness to try new things.

"Of course those things are intangible and impossible to measure," he added. "PD is rich with a different kind of data. Doing this took courage and faith, and those things can seem illogical and fuzzy. But I believe those things are what our personal service excellence is all about."

Lori Jens-Alran, director, medical surgical nursing, offers another thought about the influence of data. "People love facts," she said. "Then they know what's the right thing do to. It becomes black and white. We've seen CNAs (certified nursing assistants) who will hand a gown to a physician, and the physician will put it on. That's culture change."

Unseen changes were taking place through out the organization. Joanie Schneider, inpatient surgical RN and Jennifer Mellgren-Blackford say increased flow of quantitative data and information about MRSA have increased participation among all employee groups and expanded infection control practices and conversations well beyond the nursing staff. "I see basic infection control practices happening in housekeeping, because people have more understanding. Nurses used to defer to doctors, and let doctors tell people about infection control. But now more people are trying and succeeding to be a part of the Infection Control effort," observed Ms. Schneider. Ms. Mellgren-Blackford noted unit clerks collaborated by creating new signs for isolation and infection control in patient areas. Chris Nightingale, RN, a member of the IC team, sums up: "We encourage people to show and use what they know."

Engaging everyone in the environment was vital. PD MRSA coaches Monique Sternin and Keith McCandless came to Billings Clinic in late 2006, sitting in on several focus group interviews involving hospital staff from all walks—nurses, doctors, patients, custodians, van drivers, pastors, lab technicians—to solicit all kinds of ideas for preventing and controlling MRSA. During these sessions, questions included: How do you know your patient has MRSA? In your own practices, what do you do to prevent spreading MRSA to other patients or staff? What prevents you from practicing this all the time? Is there anyone you know who has already found solutions? Soon, some staffers were beginning to provide some "micro solutions" to the big problem of controlling MRSA. These focused discussions were called "discovery and action dialogues" (DADs) because of the action-oriented outcomes that they yielded.

"However, we made limited progress with DADs," noted Ms. Iversen, because they often turned into "conversations that focused only on barriers without solutions."

Monique Sternin reflects on the course of the continuing journey. "Billings has come a long way on its own," she observed. "It was not like that initially. In fact I remember a Billings visit a few months after the launch, some time in late 2006. I was with Keith McCandless. It seemed not much had happened in those six months as far as implementing PD as Billings was heavily involved at that time in earning its Magnet status and in conducting a MRSA prevalence study. Also, they were struggling with what PD was.

> "Life is made up of a series of judgments on insufficient data, and if we waited to run down all our doubts, it would flow past us."
>
> –Learned Hand, American judge and philosopher

"I remember Keith and me sitting in a room with frontline workers and the body language was telling us a lot. People had their arms crossed. Not many smiles. And someone even referred to the PD enthusiasts within Billings as the 'MRSA Gestapo'. I was telling myself no, no, this is not what PD is about, but it was important to not be prescriptive to those who were trying to implement PD."

"Education is not the piling on of learning, information, data, facts, skills, or abilities – that's training or instruction—but is rather making visible what is hidden as a seed."
–Thomas More, sixteenth century Renaissance scholar

Ms. Iversen and her team felt that staff was relying too heavily on the Infection Control team to find the answers to solve the MRSA problem, and that the team's "over helping" kept others from owning solutions.

Coach Joelle Everett recalled: "In spring 2007, Nancy and her team had laid the groundwork, but too few frontline people were involved. When Keith and I arrived for a visit, the team greeted us with a chorus of 'help us not to help so much'!"

In earlier discussions, staff wanted a safe place to practice infection control procedures—setting up an isolation room, donning gowns and gloves without contaminating them and then removing them safely, and handling difficult conversations. Ms. Iversen planned to have these practice sessions in an empty patient room. Keith McCandless suggested improvisational theater as a way for staff members to practice without a script, in the way real life unfolds. Ms. Everett recalls the discussions that followed. Ms. Iversen wanted to know the difference between improv and skills competency training. She suspected skills training wasn't consistent with PD.

"It was an important turning point," Ms. Everett said. "The core team had really grasped the essential difference, and was struggling with how to implement the new way."

The idea of introducing Improvisation Theater was born.

Acting One's Way....[xxi]

"How do I tell patients that they have MRSA accurately and with empathy?" asked a less experienced nurse.

"I like to tell them they are infected with a *Staph* germ that has become resistant to a common class of antibiotics. I also emphasize the fact that now that we have a culture result, we now know what is causing the infection so we can treat it," another nurse said.

That snatch of back-and-forth dialogue was one of thousands of new conversations that occurred at Billings Clinic as front-line health workers from various units got together to share insights on how to thwart MRSA infections. Remarkably, these deadly serious conversations about simultaneously managing infections and patient's feelings occurred in playful, theater-like settings.

"Improvisational play takes the edge away from difficult conversations, creating a safe space to discover possibilities that may not be initially obvious" noted Coach McCandless, the brains behind this guerilla theater exercise.

Lights, Camera, Action:
Rehearsing for Change

Ms. Iversen, who served as Mr. McCandless' co-conspirator, explained: "We know knowledge alone does not change behavior. We wanted to create experiences where people learn for themselves, discover solutions, and have a safe place to practice."

Improvisational (Improv) theater provides a space for rehearsal, especially for those who wish to experiment with new ways of addressing intractable problems. Improv's intellectual roots go back to the Theater for the Oppressed (TO) movement started by Brazilian theater-activist, Augusto Boal, who, accidentally, hit upon the idea of theater as a space for rehearsing action. One afternoon in the early 1960s, when Boal and his troupe were presenting the struggle of Brazilian peasants using fake guns as props, the peasants in the audience surrounded Boal after the performance and said:

"That was a great idea! Where are the rifles?! Let's go and take over!"[xxi] The peasants thought Boal was serious about starting a revolution. Reflecting on this incident, Boal realized that theater was not only a portrayal of revolution, but also represented a rehearsal for revolution. That is, the theatrical act by itself is a conscious intervention, a rehearsal for social action based on a collective analysis of shared problems.[xxii]

Chris Nightingale, RN, CIC, quality specialist, infection control, summarized the collective wisdom that emerged from the MRSA improv. "Various employees talked about their solutions for taking food trays out of rooms for patients in isolation. Some suggested the use of disposable food trays, however, one employee spoke up and shared her experience that if you want patients to feel unwanted, like pariahs, give them a cardboard tray with cold food. So, we didn't do that. We began brainstorming other ways to address the problem until a simple solution emerged." The nurse wipes the bottom and edges of the tray with anti-bacterial wipe

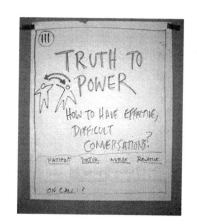

"Truth to Power: How to have effective, difficult conversations when colleagues are not practicing safely.

and hands it to someone outside the room." He who is clean, can receive the tray.

Front-line workers from multiple units, emphasized over and over again that: "The improvs were a fun refreshing way of learning. It was not another lecture, or briefing, and just right for an adult learner. The role-plays provided a continuous stream of 'aha' moments."

In one of the improvs, a nurse asked: "How does one avoid contamination if one had to hold a MRSA patient?" A colleague responded: "I put a clean bath blanket or a sheet between myself and the patient. It serves as an effective barrier."

Katherine Gowan, an RN in inpatient surgical who joined the PD MRSA effort early, describes the extraordinary opportunities for discovery when people learn together. She remembers one improv in which a staffer said she never removed her gloves and hadn't realized she should. Another hadn't realized that it was OK to change gloves in a patient's room if they became contaminated there. "We came to realize that nothing will really change until you act your way through it," she said. "That was big."

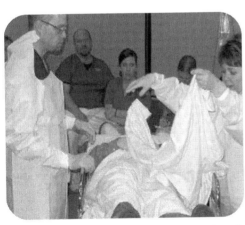

Curtis Ferrin, RN, inpatient surgical and Christy Baxter, RN, CV surgery Improv "Aha!": Unfolding a sheet to serve as MRSA barrier

More than 50 improv sessions were conducted by the end of 2007, involving over 500 Billings Clinic frontline staff. The dozens of improv scenarios explored practical matters such as preparing a room for a

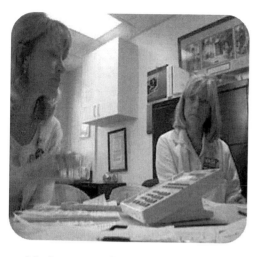

Ms. Iversen and Ms. Mellgren-Blackford make casting calls.

MRSA patient, how to transport an infected patient within the hospital, how to deal with rehab patients who are not exclusively room-bound, and how to wear and dispose protective gear safely. The improv scenes were proposed by different units, including several from the PD MRSA Prevention Partnership at Billings Clinic, a multidisciplinary in-house team to curb the spread of deadly pathogens. Ms. Iversen and Ms. Mellgren-Blackford made the casting calls, inviting people from various units, and worked with PD/MRSA coach McCandless, to improvise role-play scenes and scenarios.

During one improv, a nurse asked: "How do I make sure that the narcotic key is clean when I am in isolation room?" The solution from a colleague: "Put it on a disinfectant wipe on the pull-out shelf of the isolation cart inside the room. Then use the wipe to clean the keys when leaving the room."

Another nurse told of a MRSA patient who did not understand the reasons for his isolation. He thought he had to be separated from others because his work in a landfill made him dirty. This painful story reinforced the importance of educating patients more effectively about the reasons for isolation.

The improvs made "the invisible visible," Carlos Arce said. In one of the improvs, a physician, while examining a patient's leg wound that was oozing brown goo, paused to shake hands with the patient's fam-

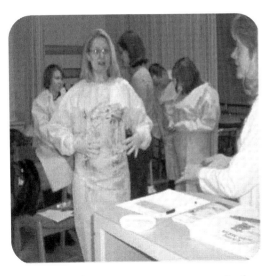

Tonda Thomas, RN, inpatient surgical
Chocolate pudding: Making MRSA visible

ily, then engaged in some back patting, and resumed the examination. Within seconds, the patient's body, the bedding, the hands and clothes of the doctor, the nurse, and the patient's family show brown stains. The brown goo, which is chocolate pudding, substitutes for MRSA, demonstrating how routine human contact spreads the deadly, but invisible, bacteria.

Nancy Rahm, RN, consultant, EMS outreach, noted: "The improvs provided an opportunity to learn from the experience of others. Folks were carefully recruited for role-plays from different units, allowing for wisdom to surface from all corners." For instance nurses acted out various scripts to educate a patient about MRSA and how it is transmitted. One of the participants later reflected, "Hearing how other people handled this difficult conversation was very helpful. It helped me think of the right words to use to empower a patient in contrast to scaring them."

In another improv, a lab technician noted that MRSA can live on fabric and environmental surfaces for up to 30 days. That was a sobering surprise for many. In another one Chris Nightingale emphasized: "The anti-bacterial gel is more effective against MRSA than a traditional soap and water hand wash." In another one, Peg Hubley shared: "I always wash hands in front of the patients, and encourage them to do so at the start of every appointment."

During December 2007 and January2008, another Billings Clinic-wide "improv festival" was launched, building on the success of the previous rounds. Several participants emphasized the cumulative learning that happened with improvs, leading to richer insights with the passage of time. As Jennifer Leachman, physical therapist, noted: "What one learned in one session, could be passed on in the successive ones, including the precise language to convey it." Kristianne Wilson, vice president for strategic development, recalled: "The energy, momentum, and learning from the improvs kept spiraling up."

"Look into the abyss and the abyss looks back at you."

–Friedrich Nietzsche, nineteenth century German philosopher

Will physicians take part in improvs? "Don't even try," said Dr. Graham, in mock horror. "You'd have a flood toward the door." He adds that the whole idea is too emotional, inefficient, and few physicians would see the need. Dr. Saberhagen has not participated, but she has watched, and been impressed. "I'd like doctors to watch improvs. If they could see the nurses playing the role of physicians, they would see how we are perceived, and that is very powerful," she said. "It's a view we don't often get. We don't see how nurses, other staff members, and patients perceive what we are doing."

How do improvs fit in with the principle tenets of the Positive Deviance approach?" we ask Carlos Arce.

Mr. Arce responds thoughtfully: "Improvs and PD go hand-in-glove—improvs are about 'acting one's way into a new way of thinking.' Improvs provide a safe space where the unspoken could be spoken, where the un-shown could be shown. The stage is a space of experimentation, with no sharp edges."

Preventing Infections
by Changing Relationships^{xxiii}

Several Billings Clinic staff members have had close personal encounters with MRSA and their harrowing experiences inject realism and heightened empathy into the MRSA issue. Chris Stevens, vice president for information technology, talked about his wife, who had undergone back surgery: "She was recovering at home and doing OK. Then within a matter of two to three hours, her conditioned worsened. She was rushed to hospital and diagnosed with a MRSA infection. Further, we learned that she was allergic to the medication that she was prescribed. A $5,000 bill turned into $50,000, and added six weeks of recovery time. She was a MRSA carrier; so if prior to her surgery, she was swabbed in the nose, all this suffering could have been avoided."

Jeanne Lambeth, an emergency department RN, contracted MRSA on her left leg when she had surgery to replace both knees. She lost 60 pounds in seven weeks and was out of work for two months. Her medical bills were an additional $50,000 to treat her infection. "Initially, I was angry. This didn't have to happen," she said. "I wondered did one of my care givers fail to wash their hands?" Ms. Iversen learned about Ms. Lambeth in a medical records review, and soon they were working together. "I've talked to large groups, I've talked to nurses, and made a tape on what this really costs, financially, physically, emotionally," Ms. Lambeth says. She still works in the emergency department, and is adamant about hand hygiene and an ardent advocate for patient safety. She insists: "If you don't wash your hands, don't touch a patient."

"What explains the recent drops in MRSA infections at Billings?" we ask Nick Wolter, the affable physician-CEO of Billings Clinic.

"There are obviously many reasons," Dr. Wolter notes. "However, the recent declines are less about implementing new technical solutions …. and more about improved interactions between people ….

Infections are being prevented at Billings Clinic by changing relationships."

* * *

In the late nineteenth century, Émile Durkheim,[xxiv] the father of sociology,[xxv] argued that social phenomena (such as civic participation, protest and resistance, or neighborhood cohesion) arise when interactions between individuals create a reality that can no longer be accounted for by the attributes of individual actors.

The nature, scope, and quality of the relationship between interacting agents in a social system influence the degree of social order, stability, or health of a system. In that sense, MRSA infections can be viewed as a result of a deterioration in the quality of human interactions. If a patient, a family member, or physician assistant does not have the courage to tell a doctor to wash hands before beginning an examination, and if physicians and other care-givers don't do it, MRSA wins. However, if the relationship between them allows for such a conversation, then MRSA can be defeated. In this light, Nick Wolter's statement about infections being "prevented by changing relationships" takes on a profound meaning.

How have relationships changed at Billings Clinic since the PD MRSA initiative got underway in 2006? Examples vary, but the consensus seems to be "yes." Ruth Senn, an LPN in inpatient surgical, says improvs increased conversations and empathy about the roles of others. She played an RN and a food service worker in different plays, and others who acted out other jobs echo her view. "There's a PD atmosphere on our floor now," Ms. Senn observes. "We interact as a team. We got the germ buster of the month award."

Ms. Harakal, the ICU manager, said ICU nurses have always had close working relationships with ICU physicians: "Once our intensivists were on board they were able to influence other groups." Ms. Block, the ICU clinical coordinator, says the work has generated increased bonding and camaraderie. "With MRSA, there's always a story," she observed. "And for every story you think of, there are five or six more. When you can have stories and a face with a situation, it emphasizes the importance, and it sinks in and becomes a lot more personal."

Social network maps[xxvi] can provide insights on how changing human relationships can contribute to MRSA prevention and control. June Holley, an expert in social network analysis, prepared network maps to understand the shift in relationships at Billings Clinic. By surveying some 300-plus employees involved in MRSA prevention work and plotting their shifting patterns of interaction over time, Holley demonstrated that connectivity increased significantly both between and among the various hospital units: More people were having more conversations about MRSA prevention and control within and across units, and more cross-unit collaborations were occurring to rope in MRSA.

"Networks are about patterns of relationships," Ms. Holley explained. "People are actually building relationships as they work together. New ideas about MRSA prevention and control are spreading through these new relational patterns, and people are continually coming up with new actions to respond to MRSA."

The three social network maps that follow present a graphic illustration of how relationships have changed at Billings Clinic in the past few years. The first network map is a baseline map, which plots the relationships based on employee responses to the following question: *Before the fall of 2006 (the PD MRSA kickoff event), with whom did you work on MRSA elimination efforts?*

The baseline network map to a large extent displays a hub and spoke structure. The three major hubs at the center are individuals who work in infection control and safety. Most individuals interact with the hub but not with each other.

The second network map represents a collaboration map, which plots the employee responses to the following question: *With whom have you worked since the fall of 2006 (the PD MRSA kickoff event) on MRSA elimination efforts?*

The collaboration network map shows the emergence of a larger core group of individuals involved in MRSA prevention (including representatives of administration and ancillary units), going beyond the few individuals responsible for infection control and patient safety. The various units (as evidenced by different nodes) are more networked within themselves and with the core, but not to the same extent with other units.

The third network map represents a potential collaboration map, which plots the employee responses to the following question: *Thinking of the future, who else could you work with to advance the MRSA elimination efforts?*

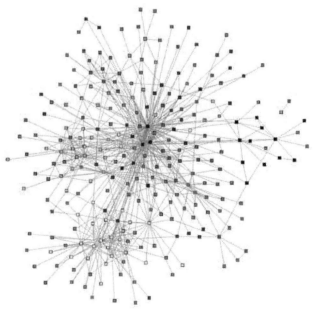

Baseline social network map

The potential collaboration network for MRSA prevention at Billings map shows a dense core and a visible periphery. As June Holley explains, such a network map represents an ideal "smart network:" a tight core, that is, dense internal connections where people have experience working with each other, and a periphery, that is, loosely connected exterior that reaches out to other groups, brings in new ideas, people and resources.[xxvi] In essence, the potential collaboration network map at Billings shows multiple cores connected to each other by their *peripheries*.

In studying the maps with her team, Ms. Iversen found several "unlikely suspects"—people who were highly connected with others and served as a resource, but who were not apparently visible as leaders. For instance, Kayla Matkin and Sarah Leland, both young oncology nurses in Inpatient Medical, emerged as "go to people." Ms. Leland developed information pocket cards so that nurses could have small

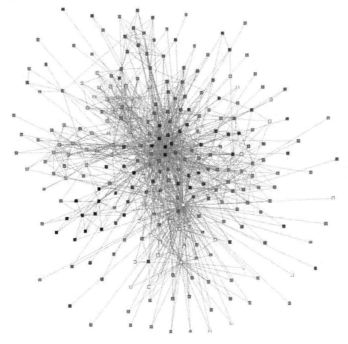

Collaboration social network map

reference cards with talking points about MRSA. Her initiative brought her in contact with other nurses on other units, making her a hub of connectivity. This knowledge allowed Ms. Iversen and her colleagues to determine who they should "especially support, draw more into the MRSA prevention initiative, and tap for influence."

Another surprise was Judy Reiland, a housekeeper in the Intensive Care Unit. She was known as a shy, quiet person, yet she was having conversations about MRSA with people on her own and other units, including physicians.

Ms. Iversen recalled "In 2006, there had been an outbreak of VRE, a highly resistant strain of bacteria. An ICU patient in one room had it, and then a patient who occupied the same room just after the first patient left got it. Ms. Reiland, who had cleaned the first room, wondered if she could have been responsible." She eagerly pursued information on cleaning and eradicating pathogens, and now she is actively sought for her expertise in cleaning and preparing isolation rooms.

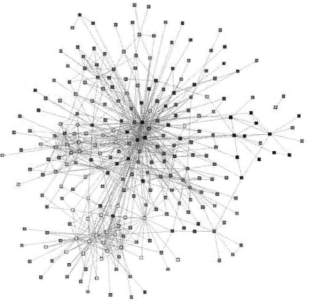

Potential collaboration network

The network maps also show the value that personal relationships bring to Billings Clinic's MRSA prevention initiative. For instance, Jennifer Mellgren-Blackford from infection control previously worked closely[xxvii] with individuals in the Billings Clinic lab, who are now responsible for the increased MRSA testing. Her colleague Nancy Iversen emphasized: "Instead of complaining about their burgeoning MRSA work load, our lab colleagues when asked to jump, ask *how high*."

Since May, 2008, when Ms. Holley prepared the network maps, representatives of all units at Billings have had several opportunities to study them. When we visited Billings Clinic in early June 2008, five large wall poster network maps were prominently displayed, and coaches Keith McCandless and Joelle Everett facilitated small group discussions to interpret the maps. The purpose of these conversations: to spur more within unit connections and cross- collaboration on MRSA prevention.

"What value do the social network maps hold for Billings in its quest to eliminate MRSA?" we ask Nancy Iversen.

She responds: "We hope to use them for forward strategic planning: figure out who are not yet involved, and how to get to them. For instance, the network maps show relatively few physicians as leaders in MRSA prevention work. We need to work with them more closely, bringing more and more of them aboard." About 20 physicians showed up in initial maps, indicating they were viewed by others as approachable resources.

"How has the role of the infection control unit changed since the PD/MRSA initiative got underway?" we ask Ms. Iversen.

Ms. Iversen's eyes glow: "The network maps tell us that we are moving toward building resilience within Billings Clinic, so that we are not dependent on a few individuals in infection control for MRSA prevention."

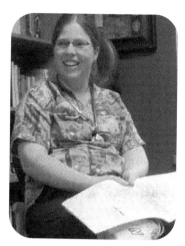

Sarah Leland, RN,
inpatient medical,
studying the network map

Coach McCandless agrees: "Those in infection control – Nancy, Jennifer, and Chris — had the most to learn — or, more accurately, to unlearn, because they kept wanting to teach the staff what to do. Managers and experts have to let some of the control go."[xxxi]

"Billings Clinic is building resilience by 'letting go,'" we muse.

When we tell the infection control team that CEO Nick Wolter said that Billings Clinic is "preventing MRSA infections by changing relationships," Ms. Iversen responded: "The network maps graph the changing patterns of interaction between human beings, and that's how work really gets done."

Kellee Fisk, vice president, people resources added: "We, at Billings Clinic, have recognized that most intractable problems dealing with patient safety are behavioral, cultural, and relational. The rising tide of improved relationships lifts all boats."

The lesson from Billings Clinic: *Infections can be prevented by changing relationships.*

Visible Changes @ Billings

"What are some visible signs of change at Billings Clinic since the PD MRSA initiative got underway?" we ask.

Dr. Bob Merchant noted: "Dr. Fairfax stopped wearing a tie. Ties transmit MRSA. Now the rest of us don't wear ties."

"How did that happen?"

"Some med students cultured ties and they found all kinds of organisms. So we have gotten rid of the neckties, white coats, and long sleeves."

Ms. Fisk noted: "Also, more visible are GelSan dispensers, isolation carts, and routine scrubbings of equipment in hallways."

"I'm an ID (infectious disease) doc," said Dr. Saberhagen, "and I wash my hands now more than I ever have in my entire career."

"What else has changed since you began fighting MRSA?"

If not entirely visible, one can sense more "shared governance" at Billings Clinic, observed Chris Nightingale: "Most staff now actively take responsibility for MRSA prevention and control. And because the staff co-created and own the solutions, they comply with them."

Another palpable change at Billings Clinic is with respect to how infection-control data is collected, shared, and acted upon. The hand hygiene data is observed anonymously, and then the staff in each unit receives a graph documenting their observed performance. So, now there is more self and peer-regulation of hand hygiene procedures.

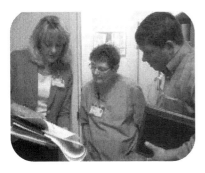

Unusual suspect Judy Reiland (center).

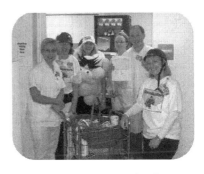

The Microbiology and Infection Prevention Team during Hand Hygiene Week

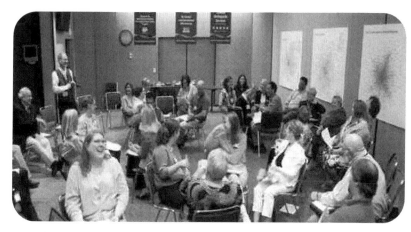

Keith McCandless (standing) facilitates a small group discussion on network maps

Further, members of the infection control team regularly compile numbers on MRSA prevalence, infections, and transmissions and share widely with staff in other units. "People now realize those numbers aren't dull statistics. They are people," says Joanie Schneider, RN. With this orientation, a CNA can now walk up to a doctor and hand over a gown. "She can do so not to question authority, but as it is in the best interests of patient safety."

The feed forward and feedback loops associated with the regularly collected MRSA data have increased staff involvement, noted Nancy Iversen: "When they see the data they see the difference their actions make."

At one point, physicians worried that patients in isolation received less care. Nurses disagreed, saying they planned more and stayed in isolation rooms longer. They also decided to gather data on the question. Sarah Leland, RN on inpatient medical, conducted a time study comparing the amount of nursing time and frequency of nursing visits for patients who are in isolation and for patients not in isolation.

"We found that isolation patients get comparable care to a non-isolation patient. The isolation patient received a total of one hour, three

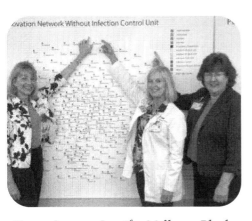

Nancy Iversen, Jennifer Mellgren-Black-ford, and Chris Nightingale of Infection Prevention & Control: 'Letting go' to build resilience

minutes and four seconds of care in an eight hour period. The non-isolation patient received a total of 47 minutes and 23 seconds of care in the same eight hour period. However, the two different patients received a different amount of visits by hospital employees. The isolation patient was seen by a care provider 12 times during eight hours, while the non-isolation patient was seen 21 times during the same period. During the study we also observed that it takes an average of 20-50 seconds to put on proper personal protective equipment or what we call PPE."

Nurse Dania Block emphasized: "We're not getting as much push-back from doctors as we used to. That is a definite change."

Mark Rumans, MD, talked about his greatly increased mindfulness about hygiene adherence protocols: "A few months ago, I went into a MRSA room, not having seen the isolation sign. I had not gowned and gloved. After coming out of the room, I re-

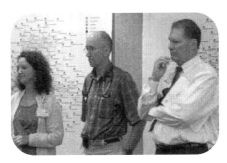

Ginny Mohl, MD, Walt Fairfax, MD (center) not wearing a tie and in short sleeves. Most who wear ties and full sleeves are administrators: COO, Jon Ness (Right).

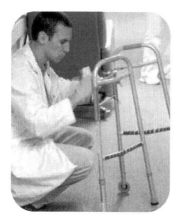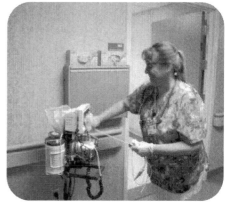

David Allred, rehab services (left) Lynn Essex, RN, inpatient medical (right), taking time to stop MRSA by disinfecting shared patient care equipment. Scrubbings are now routine in Billings Clinic hallways.

alized my mistake. I apologized to the nurse, telling her how I missed the isolation sign."

Added Ms. Iversen: "The conversation between Dr. Rumans and the nurse lead to the re-design of the isolation sign and its placement location, so it could not be missed. Christy Baxter, RN, quality specialist, infection control helped prepare new isolation signs: A STOP sign that was very visible, and specified what contact precautions were necessary. Further, the isolation signs could be printed online, and families could download the information they needed about the patient's infection, including precautions needed to stop its transmission.

Several other changes are observable, noted Ms. Iversen: "Our conversations have changed, we no longer discuss infections as cases, it is important to talk about real people, not faceless cases so we can take more responsibility for our actions."

Carlos Arce noted: "PD references continue to emerge. We're exploring new ways to use and apply our PD experience. We currently have a group of folks hoping to use PD to work on a problem related

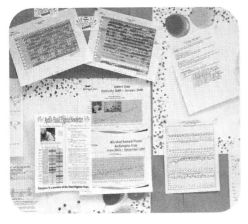

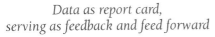

*Data as report card,
serving as feedback and feed forward*

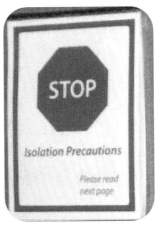

*A doctor's apology leads to
the redesign
of the MRSA Isolation sign*

to hypertension. I've been in several meetings where someone has reflected, 'Maybe we can use PD on this.' It has become another powerful option for us to create real and positive change."

Dr. Graham, the infectious disease physician, said from the beginning he thought the focus on MRSA would improve infection control in general, and while that has not been specifically studied, he believes intensified conscientiousness has to have had an impact. "This has been like a consciousness raising experience," he said. "When people ask me how, I say do you have two hours so I can tell you?" He said the lessons learned won't die. "I guess we've known top down directives don't work" he said. "I think PD is a way you get around intractable issues where you can't just tell people 'this is what's going to be done.'"

Interestingly, social changes may lead to changes in the bacterial environment. In analyzing data from Billings Clinic, Albert Einstein Medical Center, Philadelphia, and University of Louisville Hospital, Louisville, KY, three hospitals in the PD MRSA initiative that had the necessary electronic records, CDC analysts discovered a downward trend toward intervention-associated reduction in Methicillin resistance. While the data did not provide the numbers scientists need to say something has statistical significance, the downward trend in antibiotic resistance was found in the post intervention period at all three hospitals. Dr. Jernigan of the CDC explains that because transmissions of resistant bacteria were being reduced, the resistant bacteria were playing a less important role in infections that do occur, which are as a result more treatable.

In all three hospitals where data was analyzed, active surveillance of patients was practiced initially only in target units, yet the drop in MRSA incidence was house-wide. More research is needed to determine how each element of the initiative contributed to the reduction.

Another result of the initiative was the unplanned diffusion of hand hygiene awareness and the meme of collaborating to resist infection. Ms. Block and Ms. Harakal say visiting family members have readily taken to using gear available on the isolation carts outside patient rooms. They recall a six-year-old girl who regularly visited her grandfather in an isolation room being delighted when nurses trimmed her gown to fit her. She later proudly instructed other visitors on proper use of isolation gear.

The influence has extended outside Billings, and even outside the medical community. Ms. Harakal tells of a MRSA positive ICU patient who was discharged to a nursing home. "A physician walked into the room there without a gown and gloves, and he told the man's wife it wasn't necessary," she said. "His wife said when we were at Billings Clinic, everyone who came in and out wore gowns and gloves, and I expect nothing less here. And the doctor did put on gown and gloves. His wife called me and told me about it. I was so proud she had the guts to say something, and so proud she used us an example."

Truth and Consequences

In spring 2008, Nancy Iversen spoke up in a physician's retreat focusing on quality and patient safety emphasizing the need to understand the patient's perspective on healthcare-associated infections. She talked about how a patient and family had watched as one physician rolled up an isolation gown that had been handed to him and threw it on the floor, saying "I will not take this crap from a nurse." She said such acts of aggression were out of line with personal service expectations of Billings Clinic employees.

Nick Wolter, CEO, recalled: "It took great courage for Nancy, in the face of hierarchy, to tell the truth. Her words got traction for her angst was sincere. There was a recognition that change is painful, but for patient safety, essential."

We asked Ms. Iversen what gave her the courage to speak. Her polite but firm response: "Someone had to speak the truth. We were making progress with MRSA and could have used more help, which had so far not come forth."

Then after a pause, Ms. Iversen talked poignantly about her uncle, to whom she was very close, who was like a father to her, and how he died prematurely from a hospital acquired infection he got at Billings Clinic. Just three days before he died, and just days before he would meet his twin great-grandsons for the first time, he asked Ms. Iversen: Do you think if it weren't for the infection, we could have started chemotherapy sooner and I would live to see the twins?" "All he wanted was to meet and hold his twin great-grandsons, one of whom was named after him," Ms. Iversen said.

Katherine Gowan, an RN for Inpatient Surgical who was a key player in the PD MRSA initiative, had discussed her work with her husband, who is finance manager for a car dealer in town. After one of his customers coughed into his hand and then offered the hand for a shake, her husband brought up hand hygiene with the dealership's janitors. Within a couple of days, the janitors had hand sanitizers in every office, the waiting room and at the desk where customers and salespeople negotiated. She added that employees and customers are such enthusiastic hand cleaners that the pumps have to be refilled every three days.

Ups and Downs, Triumphs and Struggles

Billings Clinic's progress in controlling MRSA has not been a straight line. There have been ups and downs. However, the fight against MRSA is a relentless one: There is no letting one's guard down.

Lu Byrd, chief nursing officer, says "Identifying what one needs to do for MRSA prevention is relatively easy; however, the actions, the procedures, and approvals take time. For instance, just procuring new supplies can take weeks."

The nurses at Billings Clinic joke about the thousands of conversations they had about garbage cans. When the gown usage increased, it seemed as though the cans needed emptying every 15 minutes. Bigger cans would help, but Christy Baxter, RN, discovered there are regulations on the size of a trash can, and the volume of trash allowed. Then there were fire codes to be dealt with for isolation supply carts. Fire Marshals authorized having them parked immediately outside patient rooms, but not elsewhere in the halls. To get carts that rolled more smoothly, the hospital invested in medical carts, at $1,600 a piece. It took strong advocacy and follow-up from Lu Byrd's office, to consummate the investment. Further, the hospital began using disposable stethoscopes, thermometers and blood pressure cuffs. These disposables add to the volume of trash, so cans need to be emptied more quickly.

Nancy Iversen sighed: "We have been running on a treadmill that never stops."

Carlos Arce rejoined: "Or more like a cerebral safari."

So Billings Clinic MRSA prevention efforts have been fraught with moments of skepticism, anxiety, and uncertainty. There have been negotiations, debates, and conversations. False starts and doubts have gone hand-in-hand with triumphs and joys. However, the commitment and willingness to forge ahead has endured.

In Closing

In 1962, Bob Dylan, in his hit protest song "Blowin' in the Wind", posed a question that some epidemiologists believe signifies the present dismal state of MRSA prevention and control in the United States: *How many deaths will it take until we know that too many people have died?*

Billings Clinic in Montana is among a handful of U.S.-based hospitals that demonstrate concrete actions and outcomes to tame MRSA. It shows us how patients' lives can be saved by acting on the inherent wisdom that already exists with its frontline staff.

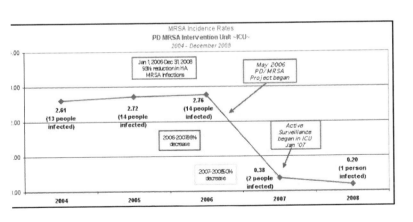

MRSA incidence rates drop to zero at the ICU

Gown Use
June 2003 – December 2008

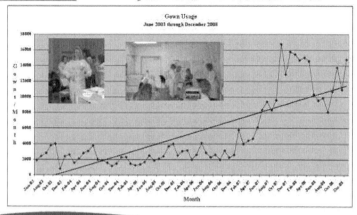

"What we're seeing here is real culture change."

When we asked Nancy Iversen, the unassuming, relentless champion of MRSA prevention at Billings Clinic, if Positive Deviance works, she replies:

"Absolutely, this has been the most effective cultural change initiative I have witnessed in my 25 years of practicing nursing. My favorite graph that depicts the cultural transformation occurring at Billings Clinic is one that shows the ever-rising usage of isolation gowns.

"When you look closely at this graph you can see that despite having current and scientifically sound policies and guidelines in place, people were not following those recommendations and were not wearing gowns when caring for patients with drug-resistant bacteria. Just when we were beginning our Discovery and Action dialogues and most noticeably, when we began Improvisational theatre learning sessions, you see a dramatic increase in gown use.

What we're seeing here is real culture change."

The graph not only documents culture change, it resonates as a reflection of Billings Clinic as part of a larger community.

"We had a sense that real behavior change was taking place here," Ms. Iversen said, "but we wanted to see something measurable. We wanted to look at gown use, which had been pretty flat for several years. I had been speaking with Shaw Weaver, our purchasing coordinator, who had the data on supplies and usage, and I asked him, *well, what does the graph look like?* He said it looks like the plains of Montana meeting the Rocky Mountains." ■

SHEA Abstract: Billings

Hospital-wide Decrease In Methicillin-resistant *Staphylococcus aureus* (MRSA) After an Intervention In a Community Hospital

Author Block: Nancy J Iversen[1], BSN, RN, CIC; Pei-Jean Chang[2], MPH; Jennifer Mellgren-Blackford[1], MT (ASCP), CIC; Christine Nightingale[1] BSN, RN, CIC; David Graham, MD; Camilla Saberhagen, MD; Edward Septimus, MD; John Stelling, MD[2]; Katherine Ellingson, PhD[3]; John Jernigan, MD, MS[3].

[1]Billings Clinic, Billings, MT, USA; [2]Centers for Disease Control and Prevention, Atlanta, GA, USA; [3]Harvard University, Boston, MA, USA

Background:

In January 2007, the Billings Clinic (a 270 bed community hospital in Billings, MT) initiated an MRSA prevention program consisting of active surveillance culturing of patients admitted to the intensive care unit (ICU), Contact Precautions for any patient in the hospital known to be colonized or infected with MRSA, hand hygiene, and hospital-wide implementation of the Positive Deviance approach to behavioral and cultural change to improve adherence to infection control practices.

Objective:

To assess the impact of the intervention on hospital-wide incident cases of MRSA using interrupted time-series (ITS) analyses.

Methods:

The intervention was introduced in January 2007. Active surveillance testing for MRSA was conducted only in a 22 bed medical-surgical ICU accounting for all ICU beds in the hospital and 10% of total hospital patient-days. Hospital-wide incidences of clinical MRSA isolates were calculated from 1/1/2004 to 8/31/2008. Incident MRSA cases were identified by positive, non-surveillance cultures obtained more than 48 hours after admission from patients with no positive cultures in the previous year. Monthly hospital-wide MRSA incidence densities were modeled using Poisson ITS regression analyses. Autocorrelation was assessed using a Durban-Watson statistic.

Results:

On average MRSA incidence decreased from 1.2 per 1000 patient-days in the pre-intervention period to 0.27 per 1000 patient days in the last six months of the post-intervention period (p=0.0001). In the 20 months since intervention, hospital-wide incidence significantly decreased by 8.4% per month (95%CI=4.4-12.1%, p<0.001). No significant autocorrelation was observed. The proportion of all clinical *S. aureus* isolates resistant to Methicillin decreased from 49% in the pre-intervention period to 39% in the post-intervention period (p=0.03).

Conclusions:

Hospital-wide incidence of MRSA decreased following initiation of an MRSA prevention program consisting of active surveillance testing of ICU patients and hospital-wide implementation of the Positive Deviance approach to improve adherence. These data suggest that significant hospital-wide reductions in endemic MRSA incidence rates can be achieved in community hospitals. Additional study is required to understand the relative contribution of the individual components of this intervention to the observed reduction in rate.

SHEA ABSTRACT:
Multi-Center Intervention

A Successful Multi-Center Intervention to Prevent Transmission of Methicillin-resistant *Staphylococcus aureus* (MRSA)

Katherine Ellingson, PhD[1], Nancy Iversen, BSN, RN, CIC[2], Jerry M. Zuckerman MD[3], Dorothy Borton, RN, BSN, CIC[3], Linda Goss MSN, RN CIC[4], Kay Lloyd[4], Pei-Jean Chang, MPH[1], John Stelling, MD[5], Alex Kallen, MD[1], Monique Sternin[6], Curt Lindberg, DMan[7], Jon C. Lloyd, MD[7], Margaret Toth, MD, John A. Jernigan, MD, MS[1], for the Positive Deviance MRSA Prevention Partnership.

[1]CDC, Atlanta, GA, USA, [2]Billings Clinic, Billings, MT, USA, [3]Albert Einstein Healthcare Network, Philadelphia, PA, USA [4]University of Louisville Hosp., Louisville, KY, USA [5]Brigham and Women's Hosp., Boston, MA, USA, [6]Positive Deviance Initiative, Boston, MA, USA, [7]Plexus Institute, Bordentown, NJ, USA.

Background:

Reports of successful multicenter interventions to reduce endemic antimicrobial resistance problems among U.S. hospitals are rare. In 2006, three hospitals (Billings Clinic, Billings, MT; Albert Einstein Medical Center, Philadelphia, PA; and University of Louisville Hospital, Louisville, KY) partnered with the Plexus Institute and the Centers for Disease Control and Prevention to implement a hospital-based intervention to prevent MRSA transmission and share electronic data for objective evaluation of the intervention.

Objective:

To analyze the impact of a multicenter intervention to prevent MRSA transmission in hospitals.

Methods:

The intervention, introduced simultaneously in all hospitals in early 2007, consisted of: 1) active surveillance testing for MRSA in selected intensive care units, 2) Contact Precautions for MRSA carriers, 3) hand hygiene promotion, and 4) Positive Deviance, a social change process that engages staff in using existing resources to solve problems collaboratively. No routine attempts to suppress MRSA colonization were used. Clinical microbiology results for all inpatient areas generated between 1/1/2005 and 9/30/2008 were electronically extracted from the laboratory information systems in each hospital. MRSA cases were defined by positive clinical (non-surveillance) cultures from patients with no MRSA-positive cultures in the previous year. Monthly hospital-wide MRSA incidence densities, and monthly proportions of *S. aureus* resistance to Methicillin, were modeled for each hospital using interrupted time series (ITS) regression analyses; overall impact across hospitals was estimated by pooling individual model estimates using inverse variance-weighting.

Results:

Accounting for pre-intervention trends, ITS analyses revealed a significant intervention-associated reduction in MRSA incidence density across the three hospitals (p=0.0008 for pooled effect). In the 20-month post-intervention period, each hospital demonstrated significant reductions in MRSA incidence density (by 26%, 31%, and 62%; p<0.0001 for pooled trend). There was a trend towards intervention-associated reduction in Methicillin resistance across hospitals that did not reach statistical significance (p=.11 for pooled effect), but reductions in Methicillin resistance were noted in the post-intervention period at each hospital (by 7%, 15%, and 28%; p=0.02 for pooled trend).

Conclusions:

Successful implementation of a multifaceted MRSA prevention program using a novel approach to social and behavioral change resulted in a significant reduction in pooled MRSA incidence, with sustained decreases demonstrated over time; results also suggest post-intervention improvement in the *S. aureus* antibiogram. These results were achieved without the use of hospital-wide active surveillance or MRSA decolonization strategies.

Footnotes

[i] Klevens, et al., (2007)

[ii] In contrast to the U.S. where the MRSA problem continues to escalate, certain northern European countries – notably Netherlands, Finland, and Denmark — have tamed MRSA. For instance, in Denmark, MRSA infections peaked in the mid-1960s – accounting for about 35 percent of infections due to *staph aureus*, and have dropped precipitously to account for only 1 to 2 percent of *staph aureus* infections over the past three decades.

[iii] According to MRSA specialists this means that a Danish patient with a *staph aureus* infection can be "treated with an old-fashioned beta-lactum antibiotic (like Methicillin) with faster response, higher cure rate, and quicker hospital discharge at lower overall cost to society."

[iv] *Staph aureus* is usually carried by people in their nose.

[v] With a population just over 100,000, Billings is the largest city in a 500-mile radius that includes the U.S. states of Montana, Idaho, Wyoming, South Dakota, and North Dakota, and the Canadian provinces of Saskatchewan, and Alberta.

[vi] From 1879 to 1881 he was president of the Northern Pacific Railway. In 1848, during the California Gold Rush, he moved to San Francisco, becoming the city's first land claims lawyer. In California, he served as a trustee of the College of California (Later, the University of California at Berkeley). In Montana, Billings and his heirs purchased many failing farms and reforested much of the surrounding hillsides around Billings with Norway Spruce, Scots Pine, European Larch, and many native species.

[vii] This section draws upon Papa, Singhal, and Papa (2006).

[viii] See Sternin and Choo (2000).

[ix] See Zeitlin, Ghassemi, and Mansour (1990).

[x] Jerry Sternin passed away in December, 2008.

xi   These foods were accessible to everyone, but community believed they were inappropriate for young children.

xii   See Sternin and Choo (2000); Sternin, Sternin, and Marsh (1999).

xiii   A Positive Deviance inquiry focuses on eliminating those client behaviors from the strategy mix that are true but useless (TBU). For instance, if a family in Vietnam is able to provide adequate nutrition to their children on account of their wealthy status, this information is true but useless in the identification of positive deviants. The uncommon qualities of positive deviants should be such that they could be practiced by others, especially those who are resource poor. Thus TBU is a sieve through which a facilitator passes the uncommon qualities of positive deviants to ensure one that the identified practices can be practiced by everyone.

xiv   The PD approach turns the well-known KAP (knowledge, attitude, practice) framework on its head. As opposed to believing that increased knowledge changes attitudes, and attitudinal changes change practice, PD believes that people really change when that change is distilled from concrete action steps.

xv   Wolter was previously involved in the founding of the Plexus Institute, a non-profit organization based in New Jersey, whose mission is "To foster the health of individuals, families, communities, organizations, and the natural environment by helping people use concepts emerging from the new science of complexity." Wolter and Plexus Institute's President Curt Lindberg had known each other for over a dozen years, sharing a common passion for complexity science ideas. In fact, in 1993, when Deaconess Medical Center merged with Billings Clinic, a physician-led-practice with Nick Wolter at the helm, it was a highly difficult transitional process, and Wolter had sought out a non-partisan mediator to facilitate interactions between the representatives of the two merged entities. The mediation, which was inspired by complexity principles of privileging open and authentic conversations between the two parties, helped overcome what was a stalemate. Curt Lindberg was involved in capturing the story of this Billings merger, especially how complexity principles helped forge new understandings and outcomes (see Baskin, Goldstein, and Lindberg, 2000).

xvi   In 2004, Dr. Wolter was recognized by the Medical Group Management Association as Physician Executive of the Year.

xvii Launched Operational Excellence (Lean, Six Sigma) initiative with training of human resources.

xviii While many hailed Semmelweis as the "savior of mothers," the medical establishment of the time shunned Semmelweis [he died in an asylum] and derided his ideas of infection control. It was nearly four decades later, that Semmelweis' strict hand-hygiene protocols would gain widespread credence, when the French chemist and microbiologist, Louis Pasteur confirmed the germ theory. While Semmelweis explained the science behind hand hygiene some 160 years ago, adherence to its practice continues to be dismal in U.S. hospitals.

xix A collaboration funded by The Robert Wood Johnson Foundation.

xx See Singhal and Greiner (2007) for the detailed VAPHS case on the application of Positive Deviance for MRSA prevention.

xxi This section draws upon Lloyd, Buscell, and Lindberg (2008).

xxii See (http://www.communityarts.net/readingroom/archive/boalintro.html).

xxiii This section benefited from Buscell (2008).

xxiv See Lukes (1985).

xxv Durkheim is especially credited with making the study of sociology a science.

xxvi The study of social networks have been used widely, both as theory and method, by sociologists, anthropologists, sociolinguists, geographers, information scientists, organizational scholars, economists, biologists, and others (Valente, 1995). Epidemiologists have used social network mapping to understand how patterns of human contact aid or inhibit the spread of diseases in a population. The well-known study on identifying Gaëtan Dugas, a French-Canadian airline steward, as "Patient Zero" for the transmission of HIV/AIDS in North America was a study that mapped social networks (Rogers, 1995). The study found that at least 40 of the 248 people diagnosed with AIDS in the U.S. by April 1982 were thought to have had sex either with him or with someone who had.

[xxvii] Along with a dense core, the loose peripheries are key as they signify "weak interpersonal ties" (Granovetter, 1973). Weak ties are more likely to introduce new ideas to network members than close ties. For instance, a group of friends who only do things with each other already share the same knowledge and opportunities. However, those with connections to other social worlds are likely to have access to a wider range of information. In essence, informationally, it is better for individuals to have connections to a variety of networks rather than many connections within a single network.

[xxvii] On account of her training in microbiology.

Bibliography

- Allison, M., What Works: Montana Clinic Staffers Discover for Themselves How to Beat MRSA (2008). http://www.reformplans.com/ReformPlans-Blog/MRSA-Positive-Deviance-health-care-quality.html

- Baskin, K., Goldstein, J., and Lindberg, C., "Merging, De-merging, and Emerging at the Deaconess Billings Clinic," (2000) http://www.plexusinstitute.org

- Buscell, P. "Pathways to prevention", *Prevention Strategist. Autumn,* (2008), pp. 41-45.

- Granovetter, M., "The strength of weak ties", *American Journal of Sociology, 78,* (1973) pp. 1360-1380.

- Klevens, R.M., et al., "Estimating Health Care Associated Infections and Deaths in U.S. Hospitals, 2002." *Public Health Reports,* 122, (2007), pp. 160-166 http://www.cdc.gov/HAI/pdfs/hai/infections_deaths.pdf

- Lloyd, J., Buscell, P., and Lindberg, C., "Staff-driven cultural transformation diminishes MRSA", *Prevention Strategist.* Spring, (2008) pp. 10-15.

- Lukes, S. *Emile Durkheim: His Life and Work, a Historical and Critical Study.* Stanford University Press. (1985)

- Papa, M.J., Singhal, A, & Papa, W.H. *Organizing for Social Change.* Beverley Hills, CA: Sage. (2006)

- Rogers, E. M. (*Diffusion of Innovations (4th ed.).* New York: The Free Press. (1995)

- Singhal, A., Entertainment-education Through Participatory Theatre, in A. Singhal, M. Cody, E.M.Rogers, and M. Sabido, eds, *Entertainment-education and Social Change, History, Research and Practice,* (2004), Lawrence Erlbaum Associates, Mahwah, NJ.

- Singhal, A., and Greiner, K., "Do what you Can, With What you Have, Where you Are": A Quest to Eliminate MRSA at the Veterans

Health Administration's hospitals in Pittsburgh. *Deep Learning*, Volume 1(4), pp. 1-14. Complexity-in-Action Series. Plexus Institute, Bodentown, NJ (2007)

* Sternin, J., & Choo, R. "The power of positive deviancy", *Harvard Business Review*, January-February, (2000).

* Sternin, M., Sternin, J., & Marsh, D. Scaling up poverty alleviation and nutrition program in Vietnam. In T. Marchione (ed.), *Scaling up, scaling down, (1999)*, pp. 97-117. Gordon and Breach Publishers.

* Valente, T. W. *Network Models of the Diffusion of Innovations.* Cresskill, NJ: Hampton Press; (1995)

* Zeitlin, M., Ghassemi, H., & Mansour, M. *Positive deviance in child nutrition.* New York: UN University Press. (1990)

Section 2
The Postscript
A Quality Cascade

This section documents the unfolding, cascading, and constant improvements in patient safety (from 2009 to 2014) at Billings Clinic, that build on the cultural shifts engendered by Positive Deviance. It also documents the expansion of PD to address other intractable and complex clinical issues such as encouraging greater use of palliative care and management of hypertension, diabetes and pain.

A Quality Cascade at Billings Clinic

As members of the Billings Clinic MRSA Partnership Council took their seats at their July 2013 meeting, they found on each chair a sheet of paper with a head silhouetted in black. Each had a name and an individual message printed on the back. The printed words were brief synopses about Billings Clinic patients who acquired MRSA during their hospitalization: first names, ages, diagnoses, the nursing units where their MRSA transmission took place, and the procedures they underwent during their hospital stay. After they read each patient's story, Council members talked about the people, the medical details, the invisible world of bacterial spread and how the interplay of practical and technical skills applied in each individual's care. What could we learn to further prevent MRSA transmissions in each unit? Stacey Dean, a Council member and a surgical nurse, took a batch of silhouettes to a meeting with more than 100 of her operating room nurse and technician colleagues. The patients' histories were read out loud and the lessons of each expe-

Patrick underwent a right primary total hip arthroplasty on 4-16-13 due to severe osteoarthritis. His past medical history includes uncontrolled type II diabetes, obesity, and hypertension. His pre-surgical nares cultures (PCR & admit / DC) were all negative for MSSA and MRSA.

He initially had persistent drainage from an open area on his incision and redness. On 4-29-13, he was given a 10-day course of Keflex. His joint was aspirated on 5-17-13 and cultures grew Enterobacter. On 6-4-13, he was taken back to surgery for removal of hardware and debridement with spacer placement.

Pre-surgical nares cultures (PCR) on 6-3-13 were positive for MSSA and MRSA. Operative tissue cultures taken on 6-4-13 grew MRSA. As of 7-17-13, he completed a 6-week course of IV antibiotics via a PICC line. He has a follow-up appointment with orthopedics to determine when he can have the second stage operation to implant new hardware.

rience were explored. This is but one example of how Positive Deviance (PD) processes and practices are "cascading through the organization" observed Nancy Iversen, director of patient safety and infection control.

Shadowing Success

As you walk around Billings Clinic now you will see the silhouettes lining the walls of the nursing unit conference rooms. You'll also find new "stick figure" graphs in the units. Each stick figure represents a patient who picked up MRSA while in the Clinic. The stick figures are arrayed by year so each unit's staff members can see how they are doing on the goal set by the Partnership Council members to reduce MRSA transmissions by 50 percent in 2013. Nancy Iversen said that so far the numbers in 2013 look good, but she was concerned with a recent uptick in MRSA transmissions. To track progress and to learn, all inpatients are now tested for MRSA when they are admitted to the hospital and when they are discharged. This way, when a transmission occurs, the site of the transfer is known and staff can

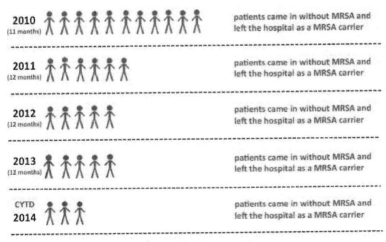

Total MRSA Transmissions
Inpatient Surgical – February 2010 to 2014

take corrective action. In the beginning of the MRSA prevention drive in 2006 only patients admitted and discharged from the Intensive Care Unit were tested. Inspired by the success in infection prevention achieved by the ICU, other nursing units embraced this active surveillance strategy. This is another example of how the PD process has stimulated continuous adaptation and experimentation, based on regular assessments of data and reflections from staff.

You can see the work of the MRSA Partnership Council is not yet done. Despite a dramatic and sustained 76 percent drop in the rate of MRSA infections—first evident relatively soon after the Council got to work and employed the Positive Deviance (PD) process in 2006—members of the MRSA team will not be satisfied until the number of infections and transmissions reaches zero. The Intensive Care Unit is close. In the last five years one ICU patient developed a MRSA infection. ICU staff members who once asked when they could stop the intensive Positive Deviance-inspired MRSA prevention effort saw data on what they had accomplished and answered their own question: "Never!"

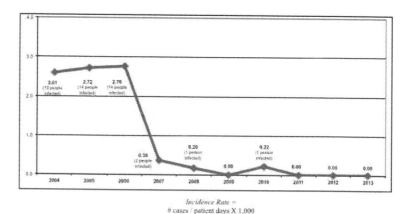

Incidence Rate =
 # cases / patient days X 1,000

Healthcare-associated MRSA Infections
Adult Intensive Care Unit Incidence Rates – 2004 to 2013

Widely known for its success in engaging staff in MRSA prevention, the Partnership Council began leading the Clinic's efforts to improve hand hygiene and reduce other healthcare-associated infections caused by other dangerous pathogens like Clostridium difficile.

When asked what she's learned since 2005 from the PD experience Nancy Iversen replied, "We will be forever different because of what we went through." She then highlighted these points:

* Peers matter.

* The process for engaging peers matters.

* We can learn from the individuals, groups and departments who do things well. Highlighting what works fosters peer-to-peer learning and sends the message we can do it too.

* Each department has a different culture and this culture matters. One needs to approach each department, each culture, with deep respect, genuine curiosity and good listening skills.

* Improvement needs to be owned by those doing the work – it's their work to do.

Other Clinic personnel offered similar reflections. Larry Severa, MD, a leading family medicine physician, noted that the PD process helped change the culture of the organization. How? He emphasized that now improvement efforts are more likely to be guided by frontline staff. When asked what quality improvement effort she found most satisfying, Beth Degenhart, the nurse manager in the Cardiac Catheterization Lab, described how infections associated with the implantation of medical devices were reduced: "All departments from the outpatient cardiology office to hospital surgery and infection control wanted to help and worked together well. We had open and positive lines of communication and a diverse group of people involved in the process."

The PD Cascade

Another cultural change becomes visible when the Clinic staff faces a new quality challenge. Now they ask if the challenge could be suitably addressed by the PD approach. If the problem is seemingly intractable, reliant on behavior and adaptive change for progress, and important to staff and the well-being of patients, Positive Deviance may help. Since the MRSA project, a number of other PD-guided improvement efforts have been undertaken: better control of pain in hospital inpatients; better management of hypertension of patients in the ambulatory care setting; and increased understanding and use of palliative care. Here are a few details.

At a 2010 gathering attended by 45 staff members devoted to bringing the benefits of palliative care to more patients and families, the first step in the Positive Deviance process - to define the problem - was taken. Here is what they came up with: "Too many patients suffering from a serious illness and their families are not offered or receiving our most complete care for the relief of pain and suffering." So staff involved in this PD effort conducted Discovery and Action Dialogues with colleagues from many inpatient units and the outpatient clinics serving patients most in need of palliative care. These dialogues led to much deeper appreciation for what palliative care is and how it can help patients and families. They also led to the discovery of new PD practices. One was a referral for palliative care as soon as a serious chronic disease was diagnosed. This led to a special effort to concentrate on palliative care referrals from outpatient clinics as well as the establishment of an outpatient Palliative Care Clinic. Before this palliative care had been an inpatient service.

Better management of patients with hypertension is a national goal because in 46 percent of the cases the disease remains uncontrolled. Primary care professionals and staff from the Center for Clinical Translational Research at Billings Clinic decided to tackle this challenge using the PD process. By identifying positive deviants and their behaviors and providing opportunities for colleagues to practice

PD Makes Inroads at Billings Clinic

Problem	PD Process Initiated	Where	Results
Hypertension Management	2008	Primary Care Clinics	43% improvement in recognition of hypertension 39% improvement in efforts to control hypertension
Palliative Care	2010	Inpatient Nursing Units and Outpatient Clinics	Increase in referrals for palliative care
Pain Management	2011	Inpatient Nursing Units	The percentage of patients whose pain was always well controlled rose from 65% at the beginning of the project to 75%

these behaviors, outpatient clinics participating in the intervention have increased recognition of uncontrolled high blood pressure by 43 percent and increased action to control blood pressure by 39 percent.

To address deficiencies in pain care quality, a Positive Deviance-informed pain resource nurse program was initiated in 2011. Nurses interested in pain management received two days of training. They learned to recognize barriers to effective pain control, ways to assess and manage pain and PD methods for improvement. In subsequent gatherings the pain resource nurses uncovered PD strategies for coping with a common problem: nurses who called doctors to report on a patient with uncontrolled pain often elicited less than optimal orders for alleviating pain.

Now many nurses report details about the patient's pain including intensity and response to current interventions. They also request specific analgesics and co-analgesics to manage the pain, and ask for a pain consultation when pain remains unmitigated. Uncontrolled pain once seemed out of nurses' control, but positive deviants showed how to advocate for patients and for effective pain management. These new communication behaviors are practiced in improvs during monthly meetings.

Since initiation of the program, patients report that pain management has improved significantly: the percentage of patients whose pain was always well controlled rose from 65 to 75.

Bright Spots

The quality cascade has reached beyond PD too. The Intensive Care Unit, where PD first took hold in 2006, is again pioneering the introduction of new improvement methods. Bob Merchant, MD, hospital chief medical officer and Dania Block, RN, ICU clinical coordinator, are leading an effort to improve care of ICU patients by strengthening Relational Coordination among all involved in ICU care, including patients and their family members. Relational Coordination (RC), which one could say is a close cousin of PD, is a theory that suggests that where people on teams collaborate and communicate effectively, important outcomes are better. Research has demonstrated that when staff members share goals, share knowledge, treat each other with respect and where communication is frequent, timely, accurate, and oriented around problem-solving, improved results emerge. In healthcare such outcomes include a variety of quality measures, including pain management, recovery, length of stay, readmission rates, and patient and staff satisfaction. Both PD and Relational Coordination highlight the central role of human interactions in effecting change, the value of different perspectives, and the power of frontline-led improvement.

At a recent retreat devoted to patient safety culture, members on a panel talked about "Bright Spots." By this they meant Positive Deviants, the individuals who helped create departments where safety cultures are strong. Nancy Iversen mentioned she heard Randy Thompson, an emergency medicine physician who was not directly involved in the PD MRSA effort, use the term "Bright Spots" in a meeting, as he explained progress he was seeing. She smiled, as she knew this concept of looking for people whose different behaviors were achieving better results was spreading. In an effort to dramatically increase involvement of physicians and staff in the Clinic's quality work, those leading an effort called "Engaging in Quality" interviewed a broad cross-section of staff, asking:

* In your time at Billings Clinic, when did you feel most engaged in quality work and what made this possible?

* What quality efforts have you been engaged in that make you feel most proud? Why?

* Which individuals or groups do you most admire for how they engage with colleagues in quality work? What do they do?

In other words, how can we learn from what's already working and do more of it? The silhouettes of Patrick and the other patients who entrusted us with their health are guides for our future. The recent initiatives and the lessons learned in the human stories behind those dark profiles are the seeds for continuing achievements in quality and safety for the people who come to Billings Clinic for their care.

Section 3
Resources on Positive Deviance

This section is directed to readers who wish to engage more deeply with the scholarly literature on the Positive Deviance approach. It is comprised of over 100 peer-reviewed publications that address a wide variety of complex social problems, including improving patient safety in healthcare settings, and a variety of other public health issues, such as decreasing malnutrition, enhancing reproductive health, and protecting children from exploitation.

Published Resources on The Positive Deviance Approach

Over the past three decades, the Positive Deviance (PD) approach to social, organizational, and individual behavioral change has yielded over 100 peer-reviewed publications. This growing literature analyzes the utilization of PD to solve a wide variety of complex social problems, including:

(1) Improving patient safety and healthcare quality;

(2) Decreasing malnutrition;

(3) Improving maternal and child health;

(4) Enhancing reproductive health;

(5) Protecting children from exploitation;

(6) Reducing school dropouts; and

(7) Boosting public and community health.

#1. Improving Patient Safety and Healthcare Quality

In the past decade, over three-dozen peer-reviewed publications have documented the impact of the Positive Deviance (PD) approach in hospitals and healthcare settings. Many publications focus on patient safety, particularly the prevention and reduction of hospital-acquired infections, notably Methicillin-resistant *Staphylococcus aureus* (MRSA). Studies have documented the use of the PD approach to increase hand-hygiene compliance and reduce post-surgical and post-hemodialysis bloodstream infections. The PD approach has been found to spur new ways of collaboration among hospital staff, broken down traditional operational silos, and empowered front-line workers to deliver high quality patient care. In complex organizational systems such as hospitals, the PD approach allows for the harnessing of distributed wisdom and collective intelligence.

- Aston, G. (2009). Fresh approaches stem MRSA tide. *Materials Management in Health Care*, 18(8), 22-25.

- Awad, S. (2009). Implementation of a Methicillin-Resistant Staphylococcus Aureus (MRSA) prevention bundle results in decreased MRSA surgical site infections. *The American Journal of Surgery*, 198(5), 607-610.

- Bradley, E., Curry, L., Ramanadhan, S., Nembhard, I., & Krumholz, H. (2009). Research in action: Using positive deviance to improve quality of health care. *Implementation Science*, 8(4), 34-42.

- Buscell, P. (2006, Winter). The MRSA issue. *Emerging*, 1-24. Retrieved from http://www.positivedeviance.org/pdf/publications/emerging.pdf

- Buscell, P. (2008). More we than me: How the fight against MRSA led to a new way of collaborating at Albert Einstein Medical Center. Plexus Institute, *Deeper Learning*, 1(5).

- Buscell, P. (2008). Pathways to prevention. *Prevention Strategist*, 41-45.

- Clancy, T. (2010). Diamonds in the rough: Positive deviance and complexity. *Journal of Nursing Administration*, 40(2), 53-56.

- Cohn, K., Friedman, L., & Allyn, T. (2007). The tectonic plates are shifting: Cultural change vs. mural dyslexia. *Frontiers of Health Services Management*, 24(1), 11-26.

- Curry, L., et al. (2011). What distinguishes top-performing hospitals in acute myocardial infarction mortality rates? *Annals of Internal Medicine*, 154(6), 384-390. doi:10.7326/0003-4819-154-6-201103150-00003

- De Macedo, R., et al. (2012). Positive deviance: Using a nurse call system to evaluate hand hygiene practices. *American Journal of Infection Control*, 40, 946-950. doi:10.1016/j.ajic.2011.11.015

- Downham, G., et al. (2012). Reducing bloodstream infections in an outpatient hemodialysis center - New Jersey, 2008-2011. *Morbidity and Mortality Weekly Report*, 61(10), 169-173.

- Ellingson, K., et al. (2011). Sustained reduction in the clinical incidence of Methicillin-resistant *Staphylococcus aureus* colonization or infection associated with a multifaceted infection control intervention. *Infection Control and Hospital Epidemiology*, 32(1), 1-8. doi: 10.1086/657665

- Friedman, S. R., et al. (2008). Positive deviance control-case life history: A method to develop grounded hypotheses about successful long-term avoidance of infection. *BMC Public Health*, 8 (94), 1-10. doi:10.1186/1471-2458-8-94

- Gabbay, R., et al. (2013). A positive deviance approach in understanding key features in improving diabetes care in the medical home. *Annals of Family Medicine*, 11(1), S99-S107. doi: 10.1370/afm.1473

- Jain, R., et al. (2011). Veterans affairs initiative to prevent Methicillin-resistant *Staphylococcus aureus* infections. *The New England Journal of Medicine*, 364, 1419-1430.

- Lindberg, C., Norstrand, P., Munger, M., DeMarsico, C., & Buscell, P. (2009). Letting go, gaining control: Positive deviance and MRSA prevention. *Clinical Leader*, 2(2), 60-67.

- Lindberg, C., & Clancy, T. (2010). Positive deviance: An elegant solution to a complex problem. *Journal of Nursing Administration*, 40(4), 150-153.

- Lindberg, C., & Schneider, M. (2012). Leadership in a complex adaptive system: Insights from positive deviance. *Academy of Management, Best Paper Proceedings*, 2012, Academy of Management Organization Development and Change Division.

- Lindberg, C., et al. (2013). Embracing collaboration: A novel strategy for reducing blood stream infections in outpatient hemodialysis centers. *American Journal of Infection Control*, 41, 513-519. doi:10.1016/j.ajic.2012.07.015

Lindberg, C., & Schneider, M. (2013). Combating infections at Maine Medical Center: insights into complexity-informed leadership from positive deviance. *Leadership*, 9(2), 229-253. doi: 10.1177/1742715012468784

Lloyd, J., Buscell, P., & Lindberg, C. (2008, Spring). Staff-driven cultural transformation diminishes MRSA. *Prevention Strategist*, 10-15.

Luft, H. (2010). Data and methods to facilitate delivery system reform: Harnessing collective intelligence to learn from positive deviance. *Health Services Research*, 45(5), 1570-1580. doi: 10.1111/j.1475-6773.2010.01148.x

Macklis, R. (2001). Successful patient safety initiatives: Driven from within. *Group Practice Journal*, 50(10), 1-5.

Marra, A., et al. (2010). Positive deviance: A new strategy for improving hand hygiene compliance. *Infection Control and Hospital Epidemiology*, 31, 12-20. doi: 10.1086/649224

Marra, A., et al. (2011). Positive deviance: A program for sustained improvement in hand hygiene compliance. *American Journal of Infection Control*, 39(1), 1-5. doi: 10.1016/j.ajic.2010.05.024

Marra, A., et al. (2013). A multicenter study using positive deviance for improving hand hygiene compliance. *American Journal of Infection Control*, 41, 1-5. doi: 10.1016/j.ajic.2013.05.013

Marsh, D. R., Schroeder, D. G., Dearden, K. A., Sternin, J., & Sternin, M. (2004). The power of positive deviance. *British Medical Journal*, 329, 1177-1179.

Patterson, P. (2011). Looking to front-line clinicians, staff for lasting improvements. *OR Manager Inc.*, 27(5), 1-5.

Sack, K. (2011, April 13). Study finds drop in deadly V. A. hospital infections. *The New York Times*. Retrieved from www.nytimes.com website.

Singhal, A., Buscell, P., & Lindberg, C. (2010). *Inviting everyone: Healing healthcare through positive deviance*. Bordentown, NJ: PlexusPress.

* Singhal, A., & Greiner, K. (2007). Do what you can with what you have where you are. Plexus Institute *Deeper Learning*, 1(4).

* Singhal, A., & Greiner, K. (2011). Using positive deviance to reduce hospital-acquired infection at the Veterans Administration Healthcare System in Pittsburgh. In Suchman, A., & Williamson, P. R. (Eds.), *Leading change in healthcare: Transforming organizations using complexity, positive psychology and relationship-centered care* (pp. 177-209). New York: Radcliffe Publishing.

* Singhal, A., Buscell, P., & McCandless, K. (2009). Saving lives by changing relationships: Positive deviance for MRSA prevention and control in a U.S. Hospital. *Positive Deviance Wisdom Series*, 3, 1-8. Boston, Tufts University: Positive Deviance Initiative.

* Singhal, A., McCandless, K., Buscell, P., & Lindberg, C. (2009). Spanning silos and spurring conversations: Positive deviance for reducing infection levels in hospitals. *Performance*, 2(3), 78-83.

* Stuckey, H., et al. (2011). Using positive deviance for determining successful weight-control practices. *Qualitative Health Research*, 21(4), 563-579.

* Zimmerman, B., et al. (2013). Front-line ownership: Generating a cure mindset for patient safety. *Healthcare Papers*, 13(1), 6-23.

#2. Decreasing Malnutrition

- Ahari, M., et al. (2006). A positive deviance-based antenatal nutrition project improves birth-weight in Upper Egypt. *Journal of Health, Population and Nutrition*, 24(4), 498-507.

- Bich Ha, P., et al. (2002). Caregiver styles of feeding and child acceptance of food in rural Viet Nam. *Food and Nutrition Bulletin*, 23(4), 92-98.

- Bolles, K., Speraw, C., Berggren, G., & Lafontant, J. G. (2002). Ti Foyer (hearth) community-based nutrition activities informed by the positive deviance approach in Leongane, Haiti: A programmatic description. *Food and Nutrition Bulletin*, 23(4), 9-15.

- Lapping, K., Schroeder, D., Marsh, D., Albalak, R., & Jabarkhil, M. Z. (2002). Comparison of a positive deviant inquiry with a case-control study to identify factors associated with nutrition status among Afghan refugee children in Pakistan. *Food and Nutrition Bulletin*, 23(4), 26-33.

- Lapping, K., et al. (2002). The positive deviance approach: Challenges and opportunities for the future. *Food and Nutrition Bulletin*, 23(4), 128-135.

- Levinson, F. J., Barney, J., Bassett, L., & Schultink, W. (2007). Utilization of positive deviance analysis in evaluating community-based nutrition programs: An application to the Dular program in Bihar, India. *Food and Nutrition Bulletin*, 28(3), 259-265.

- Mackintosh, U. A. T., Marsh, D. R., & Schroeder, D. G. (2002). Sustained positive deviant child care practices and their effects on child growth in Viet Nam. *Food and Nutrition Bulletin*, 23(4), 16-25.

- Marsh, D. R., & Schroeder, D. G. (2002). The positive deviance approach to improve health outcomes: Experience and evidence from the field - Preface. *Food and Nutrition Bulletin*, 23(4), 3-6.

- Ndiaye, M., Siekmans, K., Haddad, S., & Receveur, O. (2009). Impact of a positive deviance approach to improve the effectiveness of an iron-supplementation program to control nutritional anemia among rural Senegalese pregnant women. *Food and Nutrition Bulletin*, 30(2), 128-136.

* Schroeder, D. G., et al. (2002). An integrated child nutrition intervention improved growth of younger, more malnourished children in northern Viet Nam. *Food and Nutrition Bulletin*, 23(4), 50-58.

* Sethi, V., Kashyap, S., Seth, V., & Agarwal, S. (2003). Encouraging appropriate infant feeding practices in slums: A positive deviance approach. *Pakistan Journal of Nutrition*, 2(3), 164-166.

* Singhal, A., Sternin, J., & Dura, L. (2009). Combating malnutrition in the land of a thousand rice fields: Positive deviance grows roots in Vietnam. *Positive Deviance Wisdom Series*, 1, 1-8. Boston, Tufts University: Positive Deviance Initiative.

* Sripaipan, T., et al. (2002). Effect of an integrated nutrition program on child morbidity due to respiratory infection and diarrhea in northern Viet Nam. *Food and Nutrition Bulletin*, 23(4), 67-74.

* Tuan, T., et al. (2002). Weighing Vietnamese children: How accurate are child weights adjusted for estimates of clothing weight? *Food and Nutrition Bulletin*, 23(4), 45-49.

* Vossenaar, M., et al. (2009). The positive deviance approach can be used to create culturally appropriate eating guides compatible with reduced cancer risk. *The Journal of Nutrition*, 139(4), 755-762. doi:10.3945/jn.108.100362

* Wishik, S. M., & Van Der Vynckt, S. (1976). The use of nutritional "positive deviants" to identify approaches for modification of dietary practices. *American Journal of Public Health*, 66(1), 38-42.

* Zeitlin, M. (1991). Nutritional resilience in a hostile environment: Positive deviance in child nutrition. *Nutrition Reviews*, 49(9), 259-68.

#3. Improving Maternal and Child Health

• Ahrari, M., et al. (2002). Factors associated with successful pregnancy outcomes in Upper Egypt: A positive deviance inquiry. *Food and Nutrition Bulletin*, 23(1), 83-88.

• Aruna, M., Vazir, S., & Vidyasagar, P. (2001). Child rearing and positive deviance in the development of preschoolers: A microanalysis. *Indian Pediatrics*, 38(4), 332-339.

• Fowles, E. R., Hendricks, J. A., & Walker, L. O. (2005). Identifying healthy eating strategies in low-income pregnant women: Applying a positive deviance model. *Health Care for Women International*, 26(9), 807-820.

• Guldan, G. S., et al. (1993). Weaning practices and growth in rural Sichuan infants: A Positive Deviance Study. *Journal of Tropical Pediatrics*, 39, 169-175. doi: 10.1093/tropej/39.3.168

• Hendrickson, J.L., et al. (2002). Empowerment in rural Viet Nam: Exploring changes in mothers and health volunteers in the context of an integrated nutrition project. *Food and Nutrition Bulletin*, 23(4), 83-91.

• Marsh, D. R., et al. (2002). Identification of model newborn care practices through a positive deviance inquiry to guide behavior-change interventions in Haripur, Pakistan. *Food and Nutrition Bulletin*, 23(4), 107-116.

• Mustaphi, P., & Dobe, M. (2005). Positive deviance – the West Bengal experience. *Indian Journal of Public Health*, 49(4), 207-213.

• Schooley, J., & Morales, L. (2007). Learning from the community to improve maternal-child health and nutrition: The positive deviance/hearth approach. *Journal of Midwifery & Women's Health*, 52, 376-383. doi:10.1016/j.jmwh.2007.03.001

• Sethi, V., Kashyap, S., Aggarwal, S., Pandey, R. M., & Kondal, D. (2007). Positive deviance determinants in young infants in rural Uttar Pradesh. *Indian Journal of Pediatrics*, 74(6), 594-595.

- Sethi, V., Kashyap, S., & Seth, V. (2003). Effect of nutrition education of mothers on infant feeding practices. *Indian Journal of Pediatrics, 70*, 463-466.

- Shafique, M., Sternin, M., & Singhal, A. (2010). Will Rahima's firstborn survive overwhelming odds? Positive deviance for maternal and newborn care in Pakistan. *Positive Deviance Wisdom Series, 5*, 1-10. Boston, Tufts University: Positive Deviance Initiative.

#4. Enhancing Reproductive Health

- Babalola, S., Awasum, D., & Quenum-Renaud, B. (2002). The correlates of safe sex practices among Rwandan youth: A positive deviance approach. *African Journal of AIDS Research, 1*, 11–21.

- Babalola, S., Ouedraogo, D., & Vondrasek, C. (2006). Motivation for late sexual debut in Côte d'Ivoire and Burkina Faso: A positive deviance inquiry. *Journal of HIV/AIDS Prevention in Children & Youth, 7*(2), 65-87. doi:10.1300/J499v07n02_05

- Kim, Y. M., Heerey, M., & Kols, A. (2008). Factors that enable nurse-patient communication in a family planning context: A positive deviance study. *International Journal of Nursing Studies, 45*(10), 1411-1421.

#5. Protecting Children from Exploitation

- Dura, L., & Singhal, A. (2009). A positive deviance approach to reduce girls' trafficking in Indonesia: Asset-based communicative acts that make a difference. *Journal of Creative Communication*, 4(1), 1-17.

- McCloud, P., Aly, S., & Goltz, S. (1999). *Ending female genital cutting: A positive deviance approach in Egypt.* Cairo: CEDPA.

- Singhal, A., & Dura, L. (2009). *Protecting children from exploitation and trafficking: Using the positive deviance approach in Uganda and Indonesia.* Washington D.C.: Save the Children.

- Singhal, A., & Dura, L. (2009). Sunflowers reaching for the sun: Positive deviance for child protection in Uganda. *Positive Deviance Wisdom Series*, 4, 1-8. Boston, Tufts University: Positive Deviance Initiative.

#6. Reducing School Dropouts

- Dura, L., & Singhal, A. (2009). Will Ramon finish sixth grade? Positive deviance for student retention in rural Argentina. *Positive Deviance Wisdom Series*, 2, 1-8. Boston, Tufts University: Positive Deviance Initiative.

- Harper, S.R., & Griffin, K.A. (2011). Opportunity beyond affirmative action: How low-income and working class Black male achievers access highly selective, high-cost colleges and universities. *Harvard Journal of African American Public Policy*, 17(1), 43-60.

- Harper, S.R. (2009). Niggers no more: A critical race counter narrative on Black male student achievement at predominantly white colleges and universities. *International Journal of Qualitative Studies in Education*, 22(6), 697-712.

- Harper, S. R. (2012). *Black male student success in higher education: A report from the national Black male college achievement study.* Philadelphia: University of Pennsylvania, Center for the Study of Race and Equity in Education.

- Melnyk, B. M., & Davidson, S. (2009). Creating a culture of innovation in nursing education through shared vision, leadership, interdisciplinary partnerships, and positive deviance. *Nursing Administration Quarterly, 33*(4), 288-295.

- Niederberger, M. (2011, March 31). Clairton districts 'positive' initiative shows results. *Pittsburgh Post-Gazette.* Retrieved from http://old.post-gazette.com/pg/11090/1135793-55.stm?cmpid=news.xml

- Po, V. (2011, July). Positive deviance: Combating high school dropouts. *New America Media.* Retrieved from http://newamericamedia.org/2011/03/positive-deviance-a-program-to-combat-high-drop-out-rate.php

- Richardson, J. (2004). *From the inside out: Learning from positive deviance in your organization.* Oxford, OH: National Staff Development Council.

- Singhal, A. (2013). Positive deviance: Uncovering innovations that are invisible in plain Sight. *Kappan, 95*(3), 28-33.

- Singhal, A. (2013). Transforming education from the inside-out: Positive deviance to enhance learning and student retention. In Hiemstra, R. & Carré, P. (Eds.) *A feast of learning: International perspectives on adult learning and change* (pp. 141-159). Charlotte, NC: Information Age Publishing.

- Zaidi, Z., Jaffery, T., & Moin, S. (2010). Using positive deviance to improve student performance. *Medical Education, 44*(5), 495.

#7. Boosting Public and Community Health

- Awofeso, N., Irwin, T., & Forrest, G. (2008). Using positive deviance techniques to improve smoking cessation outcomes in New South Wales prison settings. *Health Promotion Journal of Australia, 19*(1), 72-73.

- Biggs, S. (2008). Learning from the positive to reduce rural poverty and increase social justice: institutional innovations in agricultural and natural resources research and development. *Experimental Agriculture*, 44, 37-60.

• Bullen, P. B. (2012). *A multiple case study analysis of the positive deviance approach in community health* (Doctoral Dissertation). Walden University.

• Mackenbach, J. P., Van Den Bos, J., Joung, I. M. A., Van De Mheen, H., & Stronks, K. (1994). The determinants of excellent health: Different from the determinants of ill health? *International Journal of Epidemiology*, 23(6), 1273-1281.

• Milton, C., & Ochieng, O. (2007). Development through positive deviance and its implications for economic policy making and public administration in Africa: The case of Kenyan agricultural development, 1930–2005. *World Development*, 35(3), 454–479.

• Naimoli, J. F., Challa, S., Schneidman, M., & Kostermans, K. (2008). Toward a grounded theory of why some immunization programmes in sub-Saharan Africa are more successful than others: A descriptive and exploratory assessment in six countries. *Health Policy Planning*, 23(6), 379-389. doi:10.1093/heapol/czn028

• Singhal, A. (2010). Communicating what works! Applying the positive deviance approach in health communication. *Health Communication*, 25, 605-606. doi: 10.1080/10410236.2010.496835

• Walker, I., Sterling, B., Hoke, M., & Dearden, K. (2007). Applying the concept of positive deviance to public health data: A tool for reducing health disparities. *Public Health Nursing*, 24(6), 571-576.

Foundational Resources
on Positive Deviance

In addition to the sector-wise literature referenced above, some foundational materials on the PD approach, including its historical origins, key tenets, global applications, and commentaries are available:

* Block, P. (2010). Foreword. *Inviting everyone: Healing healthcare through positive deviance* (pp. vii-ix). Bordentown, NJ: PlexusPress.

* Marsh, D.R., Schroeder, D.G., Dearden, K. A., Sternin, J., & Sternin, M. (2004). The power of positive deviance. *British Medical Journal*, 329, 1177-1179.

* Pascale, R., Sternin, J., & Sternin, M. (2010). *The power of positive deviance: How unlikely innovators solve the world's toughest problems.* Boston: Harvard Business Press.

* Singhal, A. (2011). Turning diffusion of innovations paradigm on its head. In Vishwanath, A., & Barnett, G.A. (Eds.) *The diffusion of innovations: A communication science perspective* (pp.193-205). New York: Peter Lang.

* Singhal, A. (2013). The value of positive deviations. *Developments Magazine*, 31(6), 17-20.

* Spreitzer, G., & Sonenshein, S. (2004). Toward the construct definition of positive deviance. *American Behavioral Scientist*, 47(6), 828-847.

* Sternin, J., & Pascale, R.T. (2005, May). Your company's secret change agents. *Harvard Business Review*, 1-10.

* Sternin, J. & Choo, R. (2000, January- February). The power of positive deviance. *Harvard Business Review*, 14-15.

Endnote

This extensive resource list on Positive Deviance was compiled, cleaned, and categorized by author Arvind Singhal, drawing upon resources available at the Positive Deviance Initiative website, inputs from Curt Lindberg (especially on publications in healthcare settings), and independent searches on PubMed, Google Scholar, and others. Special thanks to Anu Sachdev for standardizing the bibliography as per the citation style of the American Psychological Association (APA). A good many of these publications are downloadable from:

http://www.positivedeviance.org/resources/publications.html

http://utminers.utep.edu/asinghal/PD%20Wisdom%20Series.htm

http://www.plexusinstitute.org

Author Bios

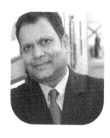

Dr. Arvind Singhal
asinghal@utep.edu
Singhal is the *Samuel Shirley and Edna Holt Marston Endowed Professor of Communication* and Director of the Social Justice Initiative in The University of Texas at El Paso's Department of Communication. He is also appointed, since 2009-2010, as the *William J. Clinton Distinguished Fellow* at the Clinton School of Public Service, University of Arkansas at Little Rock, Arkansas. Singhal teaches and conducts research in the diffusion of innovations, the Positive Deviance approach, organizing for social change, the entertainment-education strategy, and liberating interactional structures. His research and outreach spans sectors such as health, education, sustainable development, civic participation, and corporate citizenship. Singhal is co-author or editor of 12 previous books, including *Health Communication in the 21st Century* (2014); *Inviting Everyone: Healing Healthcare through Positive Deviance* (2010); *Protecting Children from Exploitation and Trafficking: Using the Positive Deviance Approach* (2009); *Communication of Innovations* (2006); *Organizing for Social Change* (2006); *Combating AIDS: Communication Strategies in Action* (2003); and *Entertainment-Education: A Communication Strategy for Social Change* (1999). In addition, Singhal has authored some 175 peer-reviewed essays in journals of communication, public health, and social change and won over two dozen international and national awards. He has visited and lectured in over 70 countries of Asia, Africa, Latin America, Australia, Europe, and North America.

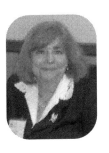

Prucia Buscell

prucia@plexusinstitute.org

Prucia Buscell is a former newspaper reporter and freelance writer who is now communications director of Plexus Institute. She is a graduate of Antioch College in Yellow Springs, Ohio. She won several awards for writing public service, investigative and women's interest news stories in New Jersey. In her work at Plexus she has written extensively about complexity science and the use of Positive Deviance in healthcare and organizational change. She coauthored *Inviting Everyone: Healing Healthcare through Positive Deviance.*

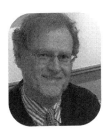

Dr. Curt Lindberg

clindberg@billingsclinic.org

Curt Lindberg is Director of the Billings Clinic Partnership for Complex Systems and Healthcare Innovation and Principal in Partners in Complexity. Prior to his current positions he served as President of Plexus Institute and Health Scientist at CDC. Lindberg earned a doctorate in complexity and organizational change from University of Hertfordshire, United Kingdom, and studied under Ralph Stacey. Lindberg has played an important role in bringing complexity science concepts into healthcare and written numerous articles and coauthored several books, including *Edgeware: Lessons From Complexity Science for Health Care Leaders* and *On the Edge: Nursing in the Age of Complexity.* In 2004 he helped introduce Positive Deviance (PD) into healthcare and subsequently served as Principal Investigator on the first multi-hospital application in the U.S. He has served as an advisor on PD projects in the U.S., Canada and South America on such issues as blood stream infection prevention, palliative care, MRSA prevention, and pain management. Lindberg has written and spoken extensively about PD and coauthored *Inviting Everyone: Healing Healthcare through Positive Deviance.*

Made in the USA
San Bernardino, CA
04 July 2015